Special Praise for *Spiritual Adrenaline*

"In everyone's life comes a time of epiphany—an event, situation, realization—that irrevocably changes life's direction. Sometimes for the best, sometimes not. While many experience change, very few are able to leverage that experience into a form and format to help others in their own personal metamorphosis. Mr. Shanahan has indeed accomplished that monumental task. *Spiritual Adrenaline* will for some be an interesting read, for others an amazing awakening, but for those with similar life situations, a life-saving treatise and blueprint to follow for the rest of their life. Congratulations Tom! You have accomplished what most only dream about doing."

Michael Bedecs, DO
Medical Director of the Age Management Center

"*Spiritual Adrenaline* is a truly a gift to the addiction recovery community. In this book, Tom Shanahan shares important information, knowledge, wisdom, and hope in an immensely readable and engaging fashion. Anyone who is interested in long-term, sustainable addiction recovery owes it to themselves to read and absorb this book."

R. Nikki Myers
Founder Y12SR: The Yoga of 12-Step Recovery

"I met Tom July 11, 2011. He came in for nutrition and exercise consultation. This is from my notes from that day: 'In my twenty-plus years of doing nutrition I believe I just met the most enthusiastic and passionate person.' I could not be more proud of Tom for taking his passion and turning it into helping others. *Spiritual Adrenaline* is a must-read for everybody from all walks of life."

Mike Foley, MS
Sports nutritionist
Coauthor, *Eat to Be Fit*

Spiritual Adrenaline

Spiritual Adrenaline

A Lifestyle Plan
to *Nourish* and *Strengthen*
Your Recovery

TOM SHANAHAN

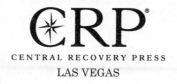

CRP®

CENTRAL RECOVERY PRESS
LAS VEGAS

Central Recovery Press (CRP) is committed to publishing exceptional materials addressing addiction treatment, addiction recovery, and behavioral healthcare topics.

For more information, visit www.centralrecoverypress.com.

Publisher: Central Recovery Press
             3321 N. Buffalo Drive
             Las Vegas, NV 89129

24 23 22 21 20 19   1 2 3 4 5

Library of Congress Cataloging-in-Publication Data
Names: Shanahan, Tom, author.
Title: Spiritual adrenaline : a lifestyle plan to nourish and strengthen your
   recovery / Tom Shanahan.
Description: Las Vegas : Central Recovery Press, [2019] | Includes
   bibliographical references.
Identifiers: LCCN 2018027878 (print) | LCCN 2018044253 (ebook) |
   ISBN 9781942094883 (ebook) | ISBN 9781942094876 (pbk. : alk. paper)
Subjects: LCSH: Substance abuse. | Twelve-step programs. | Self-help
   techniques. | Conduct of life.
Classification: LCC HV4997 (ebook) | LCC HV4997 .S53 2019 (print) | DDC
   616.86--dc23
LC record available at https://lccn.loc.gov/2018027878

Photo of Tom Shanahan by Ken Jones, Ken Jones Photography. Used with permission.

Cover design by The Book Designers. Interior design by Deb Tremper, Six Penny Graphics.

To those who remain sick and suffering either in recovery or in active addiction—I truly hope this book can help end the vicious cycle of addiction and suffering in your lives.

Table of Contents

Foreword

If you are like me, "Plan A" didn't work out and you wound up in recovery. In my case, I crashed and burned at an early age.

Broken and wrung out I found recovery. A lot of advice was made available to me, and I followed every bit of it. I attended meetings, made amends, and emptied coffee cups, until the wheels fell off. Then life got better; however, life got better faster than I did. In fact, when I put down substances, my disease played a trick on me: the obsession I previously had to use alcohol and other drugs subtly crept into other areas of my life. What are *they* doing? What are *they* not doing? My bank account. My success. The mirror. Relationships. The past. The future. All of this—a heavy heart, a crazy head—started to seem like it would never end. At that time, I thought of this as the unpleasant but indefinite cost of recovery.

But then I hit the gym. My goal was simple—I just wanted a six-pack and round shoulders. This arrived in short order. Soon, I realized something else was happening. The changes that were obvious to others on the outside, I was feeling on the inside. My mood lifted. I had energy. During workouts, I had my most creative ideas. And then, hitting the gym became my model for living. The discipline of working out consistently led to my body changing. I could see the fruits of my effort as my self-esteem and confidence grew.

I later found out that repetitive physical movement had enormous neurological benefits. I didn't realize it at the time, but there is plenty of research to back this up. We are wired for exercise. The muscles in the body are an endocrine system all their own and alleviate depression by producing dopamine, serotonin, and endorphins. I started eating better and became a competitive bodybuilder. Seventy pounds later I would see my picture on the cover of bodybuilding magazines. But more importantly, I began to feel the inner peace I had looked for my whole life. Together with my spiritual practice this became a powerful cocktail for psychic change. Up to this point, I thought my pain and frustration were inputs. But I was wrong. They were outputs. They were how I reacted to people and circumstances. The principles of recovery, my workouts, and eating better gave me the strength to process the growing pains of recovery.

I discovered the key to happiness, for me anyway. Since you cannot keep what you have without giving it away, I worked on developing a plan to share my experience. I built and opened a gym, which later became a chain. That chain grew, became popular, and the brand sustained the test of time. Much of that business model reflected lessons I had learned in recovery. For example, creating an environment that was welcoming and provided members with more than just a place to workout, but instead enabled them to join an active community of people dedicated to their own personal transformation. The lifestyle that had saved my life and given me inner peace—working out and bodybuilding—now gave me a career. Not only a career, but a way to do service for lots of people, some of whom are in recovery and others who are not.

If you've picked up this book, the chances are it is for you. I have known the author for about fifteen years. I've known him both when he was drinking and drugging and now in recovery. The difference is striking; he looks years younger and carries himself with much more self-confidence. He radiates health. Tom has laid out the tools he used in this book. Will your experience be like mine? Will it be like Tom's? Who the hell knows? Each person is on his or her own unique journey. Here is what I know as a fact and applies to everyone: A body that feels good twenty-four/seven, with neurochemicals pumping a constant stream of happiness to the brain, and liking what you see in the mirror are *rocket fuel* for recovery.

I'm good, most of the time. But there are three times I get into trouble: I get pissed as hell, scared s••tless, or ashamed of something I did. I need to surrender and get out of my head. I'm not much on prayer (just my opinion, but I think some people are made to pray and some people are made to take out the garbage). There is this little mantra I have when things get too ugly: "Universe, show me something. Show me something new. Show me something I'll like. Show me something beautiful."

Then I go to the gym . . .

David Barton
Founder, DavidBartonGym and TMPL Gym

Acknowledgments

This book has only been possible thanks to the following wonderful people and organizations: Mom, Dad, Shereen, Chris, Stephanie, Matt, Ben, Judy, David, Jimmy, Mr. Fabulous (Jude), David Barton, TMPL Gym, Mike Foley, Dr. Michael Bedecs, Saint Luke's Cathedral Church—Portland, Maine, Emile Cardali, Linda Thompson, Dr. Jason Rudolph, Kristen Davis, Melanie Albert and EXPNutrition, Nikki Meyers, Cindy Molloy, Conifer Park Staff Unit D3, Lisa Robineau, Rev. Vern Milken, Jandre Nieuwoudt, KTD Woodstock, Lama Tsultrim Yeshe, Lama Losang, Institute for Integrative Nutrition, Joshua Rosenthal, all of my Spiritual Adrenaline Inspirations, Greg Willenborg, Victoria Kuhn, Dirigo Design, Allan Carr and *The Easy Way to Stop Smoking*, David Skeist, Kevin Kavanaugh, World Gym—Portland, Maine, Scott Edelstein, M. J. Gottlieb, Gary O'Neil, Justin Luke Zirilli, Nick Lessa (Intercare), and the Buddha and his teachings.

An extra-special thanks to my literary agent, Tom Miller, who expertly guided me through this process.

Thanks also to the folks at Central Recovery Press, including Eliza Tuttelier, who first saw the promise of this book; Valerie Killeen; Patrick Hughes; Nancy Schenck; Daniel Kaelin; and Dan Hernandez.

Thank you to the authors of *Drop the Rock: Removing Character Defects—Steps Six and Seven:* Bill P., Todd W., and Sara S., for creating a road map for my recovery and inspiring me to write this book.

I also thank Soulfest Music Festival; Isaac, Taylor, and Zac Hanson; Dolly Parton; Hunter Hayes; Keith Urban; and Matt Maher and Switchfoot, for their music that makes me so happy.

Thank you to Robert Sharp, Brennon Zwingli, Kevin Robitaille, OUT Adventures, Joana Meneses, and Bodyroots for helping to make Spiritual Adrenaline Adventures real.

Thank you to Stepping Stones and AA World Services for making their collections available for research purposes.

Thank you to my friends in the Rainbow Room, my home group in New York City; and the Sunday night LGBT meeting and 7:00 a.m. Attitude Adjustment meetings in Portland, Maine.

My Story

My family has a genetic predisposition on both sides to abuse substances. Following the examples around me during my childhood and in the community where I grew up, I developed the habits of binge drinking and recreational drug use. This doesn't mean I was a bad person, but rather that I developed bad habits.

I had put these habits behind me in 2006 and moved on, both in my life and in my career. Then a host of things happened that brought the bad habits back. In 2009, I was fired from a high-profile government job after reporting misconduct. I was what is commonly known as a whistle-blower. Upset and concerned about slipping back into negative behaviors, I decided to preemptively address this issue by signing up for outpatient group therapy and committing to attend twelve-step meetings. I was not drinking or doing other drugs at that time, but was concerned I might, and I wanted to avoid that happening. Given I was depressed, I decided to see a psychiatrist a friend recommended. After a fifteen-minute consultation, he prescribed five different psychiatric medications. I was taking these drugs, attending outpatient therapy, and attending meetings.

Although I attended meetings, I refused to work the Twelve Steps and had a sponsor who never worked steps. Nothing changed about the people, places, and things in my life. I didn't drink, but I stayed stuck in my self-destructive patterns. I was abstinent and miserable rather than sober and happy. My failure to take the suggestions of those who had attained some time sober, my lack of willingness to engage in step work, and my inability to be honest about the damage substance abuse had caused in my life left me clinging to my old ways and my using comfort zone. At that time, I was constitutionally incapable of embracing the Twelve Steps and beginning the journey from abstinence to sobriety. This lasted for almost a year.

During this period, a number of terrible things happened to my loved ones within months of each other: my colleague's son was paralyzed from the neck down in January of 2010 in a snowboard accident; my brother— who's really my cousin but I've always referred to him as my brother—was paralyzed from the neck down in a skiing accident in March of 2010; and my mother was diagnosed with throat cancer in May of 2010. Within a couple of months, my entire world was radically altered. All of a sudden, I had a whole set of new responsibilities as a consequence of these realties. I was covering for my colleague so she could take time off to care for her son; I was acting as my brother's executor and health proxy, extensively involved in his day-to-day affairs. I was going to medical appointments and other meetings with my brother in Maine, traveling to Albany to help my mom with her treatments, continuing to cover for my colleague who took a year off to care for her son, and trying to run my own law firm with its many demanding clients. With the exception of my sister, no one in my family assisted with the care of my brother and mom. They had their own lives and responsibilities, and so almost everything was delegated to me.

All of my life I had been a "people pleaser" and unable to put my best interests above those of others. My people pleasing and inability to say "no" or confront other family members about their failure to help led to my being overwhelmed with demands relating to the welfare of others.

The only way to keep up with those demands placed on me and deal with stressors was to do cocaine and then drink alcohol. I realize now it was the worst coping mechanism, but it felt like the only option at the time. It worked well for a while and enabled me to be in New York City; Portland, Maine; and Albany, New York, on a regular basis to assist with treatment and care while managing my busy law practice in New York City. But then it stopped working. By March of 2011, I was using cocaine almost every day, all day, just to try to keep up. I was smoking two packs of cigarettes or more a day, and I needed to drink a liter of Jack Daniel's in order to sleep. I was a mess; my gums were bleeding from putting cocaine on them, and I was barely eating. I weighed about 140 pounds and looked awful.

Eventually, I was completely unable to function. I took a train from New York City to Albany. My sister was to meet me at the Albany station, and then drive me to Conifer Park, where I would be admitted to rehab. I had been doing cocaine and drinking on the train ride and had a major anxiety attack in the Albany train station. The attack was so bad that I was curled up in a fetal position on the ground at the entrance to the terminal. My sister called an ambulance and I was rushed to Ellis Hospital and admitted to the cardiac unit. Conifer Park waited for the results from my hospitalization before agreeing to admit me for treatment. Thankfully, after reviewing my medical records, they accepted me, and I stayed for twenty-eight days. When I left, I weighed 177 pounds.

In rehab, I could not stop eating carbs and sugars, but I did not know why. I would eat an entire basket of bread, ice cream, and lots of French fries, and I still wanted more. I drank so much coffee that I needed sleeping pills to go to sleep. I started to realize that substances still controlled almost every aspect of my life, even in the seemingly safe haven of a rehabilitation hospital. I had substituted new substances in the foods and beverages I consumed for the old choices of alcohol and cocaine. After being discharged, even though I went to meetings regularly, I hated my life. In recovery I felt stuck and thought I would never have fun again.

It struck me that the lifestyle around many twelve-step meetings—smoking, cookies, chocolate, caffeine, and sugar—was not necessarily consistent with the goal of being *in* recovery. Eventually I had to rethink everything in my life and how it all affected my recovery. I had to look at not just my habits, but also the people I associated with and how I treated my body, and, most importantly, I had to be honest about my substitution of substances for my drugs of choice. For this I had to turn to resources outside the program.

I began working out every morning and then attending the 7:00 a.m. Alcoholics Anonymous "Attitude Adjustment" meeting in Portland, Maine, where I was living. At the gym, I met nutritionist and fitness expert Mike Foley, who got me started on eating healthy and understanding that what I ate could affect how I felt and my overall sobriety. At his suggestion,

I made major changes to my diet. During my early-morning workouts I also met Michael Bedecs, DO, who explained the importance of regular blood testing and monitoring and how alcohol and other drugs deplete hormones and other naturally occurring substances in the body.

What I learned from these men became the foundation of my recovery. Yet I had never heard *any* of this information in rehab or from any therapist or at any twelve-step meeting. I realized that combining exercise and nutrition while actively engaging in step work, having a sponsor who worked steps, and regularly attending twelve-step meetings was a powerful combination.

I then heard someone at a meeting share about a book entitled *Drop the Rock*. What that person had to share caught my attention. He shared about his obsession with chocolate and how he would eat chocolate at night, trying to hide it from his family. He then explained how he came to understand that outside issues really did matter. Intrigued, I bought the book immediately and read it cover to cover in a matter of days. After reading *Drop the Rock,* I realized I was not the only one integrating outside issues into their twelve-step practice. I began implementing the recommendations from the book, with an intensive focus on Steps Six and Seven.

As a result, my body, my health, and my life finally began to change. My body, mind, and spirit at last found freedom from the substances and behaviors that had held me hostage. Moreover, rather than being sober and miserable, I was sober and happy. I wanted to share this gift with others. The lifestyle that I came to call Spiritual Adrenaline is about making conscious contact with your body, mind, and spirit.

There is a saying in the twelve-step community that "you cannot keep what you have without giving it away." The more I focus on helping others, the healthier and happier I become. That's why I decided to create the Spiritual Adrenaline program. It is my hope and belief that Spiritual Adrenaline can save lives and improve the quality of life for others who are sincerely interested in achieving happiness in recovery. If it saves even one life, the years of research and writing will have been well worth it.

I also include the stories of people who have gone down this path before. Their inspirational stories are shared to demonstrate that you are capable of anything you believe you can accomplish. Here is the first example.

Spiritual Adrenaline Inspiration: Kallup McCoy II, North Carolina

Kallup McCoy II has been sober for multiple years. His drugs of choice were alcohol, crystal meth, and opiates. He lives on the Qualla Boundary, Eastern Band of Cherokee Indian Reservation in North Carolina. Since embracing recovery, Kallup has become an advocate, raising money for and awareness of the drug epidemic in the Native American community. He recently jogged 777 miles along the infamous "Trail of Tears" to bring attention to the drug epidemic in the Cherokee Nation and Native American community.

Kallup is very serious about his nutrition. He told me, "Being on a diet has taught me one of the most crucial character traits for not only surviving but thriving in anything you do: *self-discipline*! Diet plans build self-discipline, which in turn builds mental fortitude. Eating right has brought purpose back into my life, helping me to understand that my body is a temple and to treat it as such."

Kallup runs almost daily. He uses exercise to "break the feelings of stress, anxiety, and triggers. My physical goals and the process I learn through the hard work it takes to achieve them give me so much fulfillment and build my fortitude. Exercise has a plethora of benefits, not to mention you'll be exposed to a whole new network of people who aren't using drugs and alcohol."

His advice to newcomers is to "challenge yourself with a diet/nutrition and exercise plan that will make you get out of your comfort zone and grow. When you're uncomfortable, then you're growing. When you're suffering, you're growing. You didn't mind the suffering while you were using, so plug it into a positive connection. Get comfortable being uncomfortable. It's all about the process, not the result. You learn the most on your way up the mountain, not when you get to the top!"

CHAPTER ONE

The Spiritual Adrenaline Solution

Twelve-step programs are the most successful means yet conceived to free individuals from the mental slavery of substance abuse addiction. The steps force those in the throes of active addiction to surrender, recognize their powerlessness, assess their negative and positive character traits, share their personal inventories with someone experienced in the program, and develop a road map for change, all one day at a time. The steps focus on the mental component of addiction and have helped many achieve recovery—but often not for long periods of time. For so many, the happy, joyous, and free life they hear about at meetings and aspire to remains elusive.

The relapse rate in twelve-step programs is high. The American Society of Addiction Medicine estimates that 10 percent are successful.[1] The 2014 Membership Survey for Alcoholics Anonymous (AA) estimates the success rate at 27 percent after one year and between 10 and 13 percent after ten years. For some, the steps fail to provide a solution at all, and recovery remains an elusive goal. The question is, Why do the steps work so well for some and not at all for others? There are many reasons, including the circumstances of each individual.

The solution will be different for everyone. However, for many, the lack of a focus on physical self-care and a recovery-oriented lifestyle outside of meeting attendance undercuts the benefits of a twelve-step program. Remember, the Twelve Steps are not simply a meeting-based program. Twelve-step recovery is a step-based program, and your actions outside of meeting attendance will determine your success.

Many people, once they achieve abstinence from their drug(s) of choice for a brief period, start to feel much better. Unable to cope with the sensation of feeling good, as opposed to being hung over or otherwise sick, they wind up reverting back to old habits and ultimately relapse. For still others, the steps lead to freedom from active addiction in a psychological sense, but rather than finding happiness and joy in their life, they remain stagnant, anxious, and often depressed.

Those of us in twelve-step recovery call this "white-knuckling" it. You know these types of people. You've seen and heard them at meetings for years, but rarely have heard a positive share. They are no longer out among the sick and suffering, but certainly they are not among the happy, joyous, and free. Often, white-knuckling results from the failure to take advantage of our freedom from active addiction, a lack of willingness to explore healthy new lifestyle choices, and the decision not to implement a self-care program for the body.

What does a self-care program for the body entail?

Your body relies on you to provide it with the nutrients it requires to function properly while repairing the damage resulting from long-term substance abuse. Rather than providing their body with the nutrients necessary to function in the manner nature intended, many people in recovery do the exact opposite. They rely on bursts of intense but unsustainable energy, primarily fueled by energy drinks, nicotine, sugar, and caffeine. In a manner similar to alcohol and other drugs, these substances wreak havoc on the body, mind, and spirit.

Like many in early recovery, I received most of my energy—from the time I woke up to not long before going to bed—from large amounts of coffee with enormous amounts of cream and sugar. At least one meal a day was from a fast-food place, and often two or three.

How many of you can relate to attending an evening twelve-step meeting where coffee is the beverage of choice along with cream, sugar, soda, cookies, and other snacks? After the meeting, members often go to late-night diners, pizzerias, or other local restaurants that stay open late. If you smoke or vape, add in the nicotine, and you can see that all the stimulants combined so late in the day make sleeping incredibly difficult. As a result, it's easy to linger late into the night watching television or surfing the web, and snacking while doing it. Inevitably, this lifestyle makes it easy to revert back to old behaviors associated with active addiction. Given enough time, it can lead back to the very people, places, and things associated with drugs and/or alcohol use and abuse.

Relapse Prevention

Relapse is not inevitable. The odds of relapse greatly increase when we refuse to acknowledge that what are commonly referred to as "outside issues" actually matter.

Ted Ficken, PhD, a therapist with thirty-five years of working with people in addiction recovery, studied behaviors that led to relapse in the patients he worked with and identified the things that help prevent relapse. Among the behaviors that nonrelapsers exhibited was "participation in a program of physical self-care (exercise, sleep, nutrition) and "reward[ing] themselves for successful change."[2] To avoid relapse, Dr. Ficken recommends "participating in physical exercise, eating a healthy diet, and getting enough sleep. Recovery needs to include regaining physical health and establishing a regimen of ongoing self-care habits."[3] Spiritual Adrenaline suggests a self-care-based lifestyle intended to be practiced outside of meetings and in a manner that will enhance meeting attendance, step work, and health-based types of fellowship.

Nutrition

Dietary modifications along with exercise help mitigate illnesses relating to long-term substance abuse such as type 2 diabetes and fatty liver,[4] while increasing the odds of long-term success and relapse prevention.[5] Spiritual Adrenaline takes into account the failure of mainstream treatment programs to understand the importance of nutrition in an overall twelve-step treatment program. This was written about in the book *Eating Right to Live Sober*:

> Neglect of the alcoholic's nutritional needs is spawned by and feeds on a basic misconception of the disease. Alcoholism may be an illness, these treatment programs seem to profess, but it's primarily a psychological illness with potential physical complications. This separation of the mind and the body—as

if they were ruled by entirely different mechanisms—paints a
clear picture of alcoholism as a psychological illness and allows
treatment personnel to overlook the primary neurochemical
causes of "mental" problems such as depression, mood
swings, anxiety, and confusion.[6]

Once you understand the chemical composition or substances that are
in food, you'll understand why your body craves certain foods and how
these foods impact you on a physical and mental level. Enlightened with
this knowledge, you can begin to actively decide what you should, or should
not, put into your body, not from the point of view of taste or pleasure, but
in relation to what will enhance or undercut your recovery.

In this book I'll share my proprietary Paleo Addiction Recovery
Program—or Addiction Paleo for short. Addiction Paleo is a diet high
in protein and fat.[7,8] Protein serves as the building block of the body and
represents 10 to 20 percent of body mass (depending on your age, weight,
and overall health). Protein increases your metabolic rate and helps to reduce
appetite while providing a consistent source of energy without spiking blood
sugar.[9] I also provide easy recipes for delicious and healthy treats. As you
follow my recommendations and move toward the suggested diet, your body
is slowly weaned off sugar and caffeine as the primary energy sources in favor
of protein and healthy fats.

Science has proven that a diet high in protein and healthy fats and low
in carbs will avoid spikes in blood sugar while providing the nourishment
that your organs and body need.[10] As you eat healthy fats and lean protein
in higher quantities, your body gains the ability to function and convert
healthy fats and lean proteins.[11] This should reduce cravings and assist your
body to break free of dependence on your drug of choice.

Food has a direct impact on mood and how you perceive others and
yourself. But it is not just what you eat and drink—it goes beyond that.
In *Drop the Rock: Removing Character Defects—Steps Six and Seven*, the
authors write:

> [An] area to look at closely is all other addictive practices. . . .
> Do we still smoke, binge on sugar, excessively drink coffee,
> recklessly gamble, abuse credit cards, act out sexually?
>
> Are we addicted to caffeine? Or gum? Or any substance?
> It is very interesting when we start to judge those things we

deem to be less threatening to our sobriety and therefore okay to keep. [12]

This profound observation is another simple truth: addictive behaviors are all interrelated, and none are less threatening than the others. They feed off each other. All are dependent on a lack of honesty, open-mindedness, and willingness to inventory and apply the steps in the context of behaviors other than your drug of choice.

Exercise

Studies have long proven that physical exercise reduces stress and anxiety while prompting the body to create endorphins and other hormones that help naturally improve our mood.

In 2015, Kenneth Blum and other researchers published "The Molecular Neurobiology of Twelve Steps Program & Fellowship: Connecting the Dots for Recovery," releasing findings from long-term studies into the interrelationship between a twelve-step practice and brain function.[13] The question researchers sought to answer was, "[Do] twelve-step programs and fellowship induce neuroplasticity and continued dopamine receptor proliferation" in the brain? Researchers wanted to determine whether patients' relapse rates, cravings, and other addiction-related behaviors were impacted by a failure to participate in the "psycho-social-spiritual" model provided by the Twelve Steps. The authors acknowledged "evidence that through the twelve-step program and fellowship, cross talk between the prefrontal cortex cingulate (site of decision-making) and the nucleus accumbens (site of craving behavior) is developed."[14] They also found that "those who attend regular meetings seem to adapt to recovery with a 'brand new psyche.'"[15] In part, researchers attributed this adaptation to "powerful epigenetic effects" on the brain as a result of participating in a twelve-step fellowship. *Epigenetic* means something that turns genes on or off. In this case, it refers to the production of "feel-good" brain chemicals like dopamine and oxytocin. Researchers found that those who attended regular meetings increased the release of oxytocin, a bonding chemical produced in the brain, resulting in "a newfound happiness."[16]

A 2017 study at NYU/Langone Medical Center in New York was the first to use MRI scans to prove that AA slogans and prayers improved brain function in long-term members of AA and helped to reduce cravings to drink.[17]

Science is beginning to unravel the psychological reasons twelve-step programs work and, in turn, provide evidence that just as the gym provides exercise for the body, meetings provide exercise for the mind. A November 2015 study conducted by UCLA concluded that exercise contributed to the regrowth of dopamine receptors in patients in recovery from addiction to crystal meth.[18] Although it focused on meth use and recovery, the study has broad application for alcoholism and abuse of other substances as it confirms that when provided with positive stimuli, your body has the capacity to heal itself, even after years of substance abuse. You can incorporate exercise in a way that enhances your existing twelve-step program by timing exercise around meeting attendance, service commitments, personal inventories, and making amends. By timing your exercise to supplement your twelve-step program, you maintain a positive mind-set throughout the day. For example, if you plan to attend a midday or evening meeting, I suggest working out in the morning, and vice versa.

By structuring the day around these healthy activities, you can avoid envy, resentments, and other character defects as your body and mind remain in gratitude and prompt your body to produce hormones that provide a natural high. For example, endorphins increase your sense of pleasure and enhance your mood. Although your endorphin production may have been negatively affected by long-term use of alcohol or other drugs, studies confirm that over time proper hormone levels will return. Normal production of almost all hormones will return over time if you stay committed to living the self-care lifestyle in this book.

Here are just some of the undisputed benefits associated with exercise:

- Expands the vascular system in muscle tissue and prevents high blood pressure and hypertension
- Builds up muscle mass and prevents muscle breakdown and atrophy
- Stimulates activity of fat-burning enzymes and promotes the manufacture of energy for muscle activity
- Lowers blood sugar
- Enhances bone and joint health
- Increases production of vital hormones that enhance libido and sexual performance

- Stimulates the sympathetic nervous system and increases production of adrenaline
- Promotes the production of endorphins and other positive natural hormones in the body

Just as you learned to find time to attend meetings regularly, you can learn to integrate exercise into your daily routine. Spiritual Adrenaline includes all the exercise tools you will need to get started on your journey toward physical fitness.

Spiritual Toolbox

Your spiritual toolbox involves utilizing a series of simple yet powerful tools to increase your connection to the Twelve Steps, nature, other people, and the world around you. When utilized properly, these tools are strong mechanisms to restore your mind to the present moment, permitting you to live in the now. Your spiritual tools do not involve traveling to India or other exotic locations and do not require you to invest substantial sums of money in new clothes or spiritual retreats. The Spiritual Adrenaline tools are geared to open your eyes to the spirituality all around you. I will help you find spirituality in shopping for your food, in preparing your meals, in the food you eat, in the self-care you practice while working out, in the music you listen to, and in your twelve-step practice.

Most of all, I'm trying to help you make conscious contact with your body. When combined with the Spiritual Adrenaline nutrition and exercise regime, both body and mind are developed into productive, highly functional tools that complement each other. Over time, you will learn to take refuge in your body during difficult times, rather than in food, sex, shopping, gambling, internet, chaos, or substances. The next logical step, the natural consequence of healthy living, will be an amazing sense of connectedness and new appreciation for your own body and its potential, as well as an appreciation for the people, places, and things that surround you.

Stepping Out of Your Comfort Zone

You may have heard the saying, "Life begins when you step out of your comfort zone." Be forewarned, Spiritual Adrenaline will require you to step out of your existing comfort zone and how you previously thought of your recovery. You may have been told by your sponsor, therapist, or others at meetings to avoid focusing on "outside issues." The advice in this book is the complete opposite. It's critical to understand that Spiritual Adrenaline is *not* a substitute for a traditional twelve-step program, working with your sponsor, and regular meeting attendance. Only after you have established a solid foundation in your twelve-step practice and after *at least* six months in recovery should you begin to focus your energy on the interrelated outside issues. The reason is simple: when you come into recovery you are already stepping out of your existing comfort zone. You have already shown the courage to step out of active addiction and the willingness to embrace change. You may not have realized it, but undertaking Step One and accepting surrender is your first spiritual awakening.

Since everything is new, you have to learn to pace yourself. The tendency of those with addictive disease is to want to get it all done as soon as possible. Work all twelve steps in one day, make all your amends in a week, and then declare yourself "cured." That is not how recovery works. Repeating the slogan "Easy does it" will help slow you down in the pursuit of goals you set to ensure you are not self-sabotaging and setting yourself up for failure. You did not become addicted in a couple of days or weeks or months, and you are not going to recover in days or weeks or months. Recovery is a lifelong commitment that you make one day at a time.

In addition, each of you will have a different goal. Some may want to be able to walk around the block or take a short bike ride to visit a friend. Others may want six-pack abs, to compete in a triathlon, or maybe to run a marathon. Everything in this book is customizable for you based on your addiction history, where you find yourself in the present, and your long-term goals. You must remember to avoid what is commonly known as "compare and despair." Set your goals based on what is achievable for you, not what others want for you or what others are doing.

Positive Reinforcement

Everyone starts somewhere. As you already know, breaking the cycle of addiction is hard work; it's among the most daunting challenges many people will face in their lifetime. Long-term behavioral modification takes substantial effort and dedication. No one ever said this is easy. However, Spiritual Adrenaline works where other programs fail because the motivation to continue is self-generated through positive reinforcement. This happens when you start to see your body transform while you are enjoying the natural high created by providing your body with the nourishment it needs rather than living under constant stress and running your body into the ground.

Modifying Your Reward System

If you apply the tools in this book, over time you will see your reward system change—not intentionally, but instead based upon the positive lifestyle changes you are implementing. Gulping a drink, popping a pill, smoking a bowl, or doing a line will lose its appeal compared to enjoying a yoga class, a day-trip to the museum or beach, a retreat weekend, taking a loved one out for dinner, helping your sponsee, showing up for your meeting commitment, or sharing your success with others at a meeting. Rather than rewards that undercut the achievement you are celebrating, you embrace rewards that continue to strengthen the foundation of your new recovery-oriented life. I will offer various ways to measure your progress—some physical, some psychological, and some based on your blood work—so you can find the measure that serves your needs and abilities. The key is to avoid self-sabotage caused by setting unrealistic goals. To avoid falling into this trap, I encourage you to set and attain smaller, more realistic goals. This will give you the confidence you need to keep moving in the right direction. There is no better motivation than *positive* reinforcement.

In this book, guidance and general parameters are offered. The Spiritual Adrenaline program is totally customizable to ensure you have the best chance possible of succeeding on your journey to find happiness and peace of mind in recovery.

The Spiritual Adrenaline online community on Facebook is full of other people from all around the world who are integrating the Spiritual Adrenaline program into their recovery. So you are not alone on this journey and will have plenty like-minded people to support you.

Let's get started!

Spiritual Adrenaline Inspiration: Scott R., Illinois

Scott's been sober since October 2, 1988. He is a recovering alcoholic who also abused drugs, including marijuana and LSD. Today, Scott is a certified triathlon coach and has competed in, and successfully finished, two Ironman competitions, and an ultra-marathon of 50K in his sixties.

After entering recovery from alcohol and other drugs, it took him seventeen more years to confront excessive eating. The solution to each problem was the same: admitting he couldn't do it alone, asking for spiritual help, and taking positive action. Every victory over addictive behavior reinforced recovery while lending proof of the existence of a loving higher power that only wanted the best for him.

Scott believes God enters us through our wounds. As with alcohol and drugs before it, his recovery from excessive eating reinforced that fact and provided the foundation of what he experienced as a "spiritual awakening."

Scott does not believe that nutrition and exercise are "outside issues" in addiction recovery. In fact, he does not believe there are any "outside issues." He told me, "If it affects your desire to stop drinking, then it is a central issue to recovery from alcoholism. The bottle, we are taught, is merely a symptom of underlying living problems. So are drugs. Both founders of Alcoholics Anonymous mention their drug abuse in the organization's Big Book. Other symptoms of underlying living problems include eating disorders, gambling, acting out sexually, and other negative behaviors. Steps Six and Seven address these issues."

He believes life is all about habits. If you repeat bad habits, bad things happen. If you replace them with good habits, good things happen— anything that helps him learn more about the process of surrender, inventory, confession, restitution, prayer, meditation, and service, and teaches him lessons those apply to every aspect of his life. Through exercise and good nutrition, he has learned more about self-discipline and positive self-love.

He believes exercise is active meditation. Whether yoga or cycling, running, swimming, or working with kettlebells, exercise involves repetitive actions that help him focus his mind, body, and spirit on this present moment where all change occurs.

Whenever he feels any stress, it leaves when he refuses to stare at the past or to predict the future. Thanks to triathlons and the cross-training it requires, he is stronger and better able to deal with whatever may come his way. His advice for newcomers who want to lose weight or just get in shape is to stop thinking about it and just get started. At his top weight, Scott was 400 pounds. He went to a bike shop and bought a bike. In the first year, he lost substantial weight. He beat cancer a year later, entered triathlons three years after that, and crossed the finish line of his first Ironman just shy of age sixty, after losing about 175 pounds. He did his second Ironman two years later and became a USA Triathlon coach.

Scott recommends newcomers join a gym or health club, ask for help from people who are living the lifestyle they want, and build relationships with those people. He also recommends working out with friends. Accountability goes a long way toward motivating you to get out of a cozy bed at 5:00 a.m. to go for a run or a bike workout or a swim. He also encourages newcomers to exercise and to set goals. Sign up for a 5K run or an organized bike ride and lock in the motivation by posting the date in places where you will see it routinely, like your refrigerator, your post-it board, or your bathroom mirror.

CHAPTER TWO

The Twelve Steps and More

At the time Bill W. and Dr. Bob, the cofounders of Alcoholics Anonymous, conceived the Twelve Steps, science hadn't kept pace in the context of the role of self-care and nutrition in achieving sobriety and preventing relapse. Although the founders lacked the benefit of scientific research, they had lots of common sense and their own experience as alcoholics trying to get, and stay, sober. Let's take a look back to the early days of recovery: the 1930s through 1960s.

Nutrition and the Steps

When AA was founded in 1935, there was little information available regarding the importance of nutrition and how the substances that compose food could play a role in reducing cravings and helping people stay sober. Early twelve-step members developed their own social culture around the program. Smoking was pervasive and meetings were notoriously held in smoke-filled rooms. Most meetings offered attendees copious amounts of coffee and sugary treats such as cookies or donuts. Socializing after meetings, which became known as "fellowshipping," often involved diners, pizzerias, or other places that were open late and served inexpensive food.

Twelve-step groups have a principle that they take no position on outside issues that would detract from a focus on the primary purpose of the particular twelve-step group. For example, people attending AA are there to focus on their alcohol consumption. People at Overeaters Anonymous are there to address their relationship with food. If the group's focus is not on the primary issue of concern, people will likely be turned off and stop going. Among the outside issues in the context of substance abuse are nutrition and exercise. So although speakers at meetings may address these topics if it relates to their subjective experience and members may share on these topics, none of the major twelve-step fellowships servicing the substance abuse community has ever formulated a policy with regard to nutrition and exercise.

That said, Bill W. and Dr. Bob linked modifications in the diet to the overall success of those seeking to stop the vicious cycle of drinking. In the early days, AA recommended newcomers eat certain foods believed to help reduce cravings. These recommendations were based upon the experience of others who had achieved success in remaining sober. Among the foods recommended were frankfurters and tomato paste. An early documented example was an AA member named Eddie. Eddie was constantly coming in and out AA meetings and could not accumulate more than a couple of days sober before relapsing. Eddie would frequently go on drinking binges, and when he did he acted out in a crazy manner. Fellow AA members tried to help him sober up and calm down by feeding him baking soda, which they believed would restore Eddie to sanity. For an unknown reason, the baking soda seemed to work. However, as soon as Eddie would sober up with the help of baking soda and after eating a good meal, "he'd go off his rocker again."[19]

All this changed when Dr. William Silkworth came to meet and work with Bill W. Dr. Silkworth was a well-known early expert on alcoholism. Dr. Silkworth was responsible for helping members to focus on their diet as part of their overall recovery. Bill W. recalled, "It was Dr. Silkworth who introduced the idea to me that alcoholism had a physical component—something he called an 'allergy.' He knew this was a misnomer; he used it to express his intuition that something was physically wrong with most of us, a factor perhaps causative and certainly an aggravation of the alcoholic's condition."[20] Dr. Silkworth's "allergy" theory was based upon his research into the overall health of and diseases common in alcoholics.

His pioneering research was the first to document the prevalence of hypoglycemia, or low blood sugar, in many alcoholics. He also documented the high percentage of alcoholics with type 2 diabetes, then known as adult-onset diabetes.[21] Dr. Silkworth understood these conditions were controllable through diet. He encouraged Bill W. and AA to recommend that those in both active addiction and sobriety modify their diet to reduce cravings and prevent relapse. Dr. Silkworth recommended that alcoholics eat small amounts of glucose, sucrose, or other simple carbohydrates and substantial amounts of complex carbohydrates. He also recommended low caffeine intake. Although radical at that time, these principles are well accepted today.

Adopting Dr. Silkworth's research, Bill W. and, to a lesser extent, Dr. Bob began to recommend certain lifestyle changes to AA members and professionals providing services to alcoholics. In a 1968 communication to physicians associated with AA, Bill W. noted: "We alcoholics try to cure these conditions of hypoglycemia first by sweets and then by coffee. . . . In exactly the wrong way, we are trying to treat ourselves for hypoglycemia."[22] Over the years and after the death of Dr. Bob, Bill W. continued to conduct his unscientific research on lifestyle modification.

Bill W. proposed modifications to AA's Twelve Traditions. He recommended that nutritional guidelines be incorporated into the overall AA program. The AA board rejected his research and proposed modifications. The AA board's position was based upon the Tenth Tradition of AA—that AA takes "no position on outside issues." Despite AA's position, Bill W. continued to advocate for awareness of the interrelationships among food, mood, health, and alcoholism. For example, in 1968 Bill W. wrote a memorandum to AA-affiliated physicians, noting the exceedingly high rate of hypoglycemia in alcoholics. He felt the need to address nutrition in the context of "sister foods" to alcohol, such as refined sugar, soda, white bread, rice, pasta, potatoes, and French fries[23] and how these foods were contributing to relapse in people who identified as members of the recovery community.

Bill W. also recognized the link between vitamins and minerals and medical conditions related to alcoholism such as anxiety and depression. He experimented with niacin and published three pamphlets on his niacin research.[24] Bill's experimentation with vitamins and minerals was precipitated by his lifelong struggle with depression that continued even after he got sober.

In 1958, Bill began working with a well-known medical practitioner, Dr. Abram Hoffer, to treat his tension, depression, fatigue, and insomnia. To deal with these issues, Dr. Hoffer put him on a regimen of 1,000 milligrams of niacin, three times a day. Bill noticed that many of his symptoms seemingly disappeared. Astounded by the dramatic improvement, Bill conducted his own unscientific study of thirty people in AA. He began giving them niacin and started to track their progress and their ability to stop drinking. After one month of taking the niacin, signs and symptoms of alcoholism went away for ten people. After two months, another ten people experienced the same effect. The final ten experienced no change.[25]

Bill W. became a vocal supporter of nutritional therapy as a part of recovery for those suffering with alcoholism. Once again, the AA board of directors distanced the organization from Bill's niacin advocacy. The AA board took the position that Tradition Ten precluded AA from taking a position on this outside issue. The board concluded that just as nutritional advocacy was not permissible, neither was advocacy relating to supplements. Among other things, the board was concerned that Bill lacked any medical or nutritional qualifications and so was not qualified to weigh in on these issues. Bill was given a choice: to remain on the AA board and cease public advocacy on these outside issues or to resign and continue his advocacy. Bill chose to stay on the AA board. He thereafter discontinued public advocacy for integration of nutritional or supplemental recommendations into AA's steps or traditions.

Fast-Forward to the Present

Credible recent research studies have reported that up to 90 percent of newcomers to the recovery community are either hypoglycemic or diabetic.[26] Clearly, the health concerns identified so long ago by Dr. Silkworth remain a major issue in the recovery community today. These figures demonstrate that an epidemic exists when it comes to hypoglycemia and type 2 diabetes. Research also proves that these conditions are directly related to diet and can be mitigated or eliminated through exercise and modification to diet.

I will introduce my Addiction Paleo plan at length in Chapter Nine. Addiction Paleo involves slowly weaning the body off sugar and caffeine as primary energy sources and learning to eat healthy fats[27] and lean proteins instead for more sustainable energy without spiking blood sugar. Recently, studies have confirmed that paleo diets not only provide sustainable energy, they also help reverse both heart disease and type 2 diabetes; both are prevalent in the recovery community.[28] Not only is my plan good for you, but it will satisfy your sweet tooth by providing you with delicious and healthy alternatives to comfort foods while weaning you off sugar, fructose, high-fructose corn syrup, and other unsustainable energy sources.

Smoking is another problem with people in recovery. It has long been accepted as a social norm in twelve-step communities. As a person who smoked for twenty-four years and who did not think I would ever be able to quit, I understand the suffering caused by the drug nicotine. Clearly, smoking is not recovery-oriented behavior, as nicotine does what all drugs do—it dominates your thoughts and behaviors, defines your social circles and activities, and ultimately leads to death in a slow and insidious manner, similar to the way alcohol and other drugs do.

When I visited Stepping Stones, Bill W.'s home in Westchester County, New York, I was privileged to see the actual desk at which he wrote what is now known as the Big Book. As I studied that piece of history, something unexpected grabbed my attention. Bill didn't use an ashtray, so all around the edges of the desk are cigarette burns where Bill, a lifelong smoker, would rest his cigarettes. Sadly, he ultimately passed away of lung-related disease. The cigarette burns around the desk left a profound impact on me. The fact that someone as brilliant as Bill, who cofounded AA and was able to quit drinking and inspire millions, died from smoking-related illness drove home the point of just how insidious nicotine addiction truly is. According to Dr. Richard D. Hurt, head of the Nicotine Dependence Center at the Mayo Clinic, a little more than half of all people in addiction recovery will ultimately die of a tobacco-related disease.[29]

So what may have been debatable back in the day of Dr. Silkworth and Bill W. cannot be debated any longer. The epidemics of hypoglycemia, diabetes, and smoking-related illnesses in the recovery community are real and the evidence is clear. It's up to you to surrender to these facts just as we did to our powerlessness over our drug(s) of choice. You must then do a fearless and searching self-care inventory and develop, with the help of qualified people, action steps to make amends not only to others, but also to your body. Thankfully, there are modern-day recovery pioneers who have developed programs to help. Most of these programs are common sense–based self-care programs founded by people who identify as members of the recovery community.

How Is Spiritual Adrenaline Different?

Not everyone can afford a personal trainer or has access to a local organization that offers body-mind-spirit programming. And yoga is not for everyone. Weight training and other types of exercise and/or aerobic or outdoor activities get substantially less attention. The Spiritual Adrenaline program fills that void and this book, my website (spiritualadrenaline.com), my Facebook page (@SpiritualAdrenaline), and Instagram page (@spiritual_adr) focus on the multitude of ways people in addiction recovery can incorporate self-care into their twelve-step programs.

Spiritual Adrenaline Inspiration: **Yana K., New York**

Yana K. of Rochester, New York, is a recovering alcoholic and drug addict; besides alcohol, her drugs of choice included cocaine and prescription pills.

> Coming from a place of destruction, I could never have imagined a life of freedom. Before I entered recovery, I was not physically active in the least. But that all changed when I met someone who showed me how to have pure, unadulterated fun in sobriety. And from there, we were off. My fiancé Sean, his best friend Patrick, and I started a program called ROCovery Fitness, a peer-led sober active community in Rochester, New York. We had no intention of starting a program and just wanted to stay clean and sober. We started with simple hikes with others in recovery, and from there we began more frequent and diverse types of activities. In over two years we connected with close to 1,000 individuals in recovery through health, wellness, and exercise. We have created an army of people committed to sober living and recovery.
>
> Exercise and wellness saved my life and the lives of many others. Sadly, our friend Pat lost his life to the disease of addiction

in March of 2017, two short months before we opened our active sober community center. We continue to honor Pat's life and the lives of all those lost by advancing ROCovery's mission and providing a free, safe, and nurturing environment for those in recovery.

Exercise is an antidepressant, an antianxiety drug, a stress reducer, and an all-around happy pill. There are minimal side effects: sore muscles, increased energy, increased heart rate, endorphin release, an urge to be out in nature, and a desire to be around like-minded people. When I am stressed, I know where to turn and what to do. Before recovery and exercise, I would use drugs, alcohol, people, drama, and the like to try to numb the pain and *dis*-ease. Today, I run and hike and go kayaking as a way to truly manage stress and be able to face each day with dignity and grace.

Get out there and move! Just go! Get outside, call a friend, and inspire others to do the same—whether it is going for a walk or jumping on a bike. Exercise is not just about going to a gym and walking on a treadmill. Exercise is *fun*! Look up places to hike, download a step tracker, anything. Just do it. You've probably spent hours of your life doing things you aren't proud of. Take an hour and do something you can feel good about.

CHAPTER THREE

Nourishing Your Recovery

How many times have you heard someone share at a meeting about eating crazy amounts of candy, ice cream, or other sweets as a kid, teenager, or even as an adult? When I was a young, I could finish an entire chocolate cake in one sitting. No exaggeration; I could finish the whole thing. Today, it's clear that sugar was my first addiction. Looking at it another way, sugar was my "gateway drug." In hindsight, these childhood and teenage behaviors are consistent with my behaviors later in life with alcohol and then other drugs. One slice of chocolate cake, one beer, or one line of coke—that was a natural progression for me. I was never happy with just one and could never get enough. Childhood behaviors set the pattern for my later life and my relationship with other substances.

In *Drop the Rock,* the authors write: "Many of us do not balance our dietary habits. Many of us are addicted to sugar and carbohydrates. We binge and diet, binge and diet. We have eating problems."[30] For most, their dysfunctional relationship with food revolves around sugar and caffeine. These substances are among those that mimic alcohol and other drugs when ingested, as they flood the brain with dopamine.[31] Over time, your body builds up a tolerance to these addictive substances and it takes more and more of them to replicate the pleasurable feeling.[32] Not only does it take more, but if you don't get more, you experience cravings. This pattern begins the cycle of excessive intake, satisfaction, withdrawal, and then craving.

One of your major goals after reading *Spiritual Adrenaline* will be to break the cycle described in *Drop the Rock* and instead learn to integrate healthy food, snacks, and desserts into your recovery. Rather than making you miserable, I hope it will make you feel better and look better, and provide you with all the energy you need to not only function, but also thrive. In later chapters, I will cover the foods I recommend for you to consider as a person in recovery. My recommendations are only suggestions. You will pick and choose based upon your own tastes, energy needs, and long-term goals. This will be different for everyone, so the program is designed to be modified by you for you. I also introduce you to some tools that will help make eating in a manner consistent with your recovery easy, without sacrificing your sweet tooth.

Following are the basics of the Spiritual Adrenaline nutritional program. If you have some basic knowledge you can skip ahead; however, I recommend you read this chapter since my focus is somewhat different from that of other mainstream lifestyle books. My recommendations are designed for people like us: members of the addiction recovery community. Your investment of time now will ensure you don't unintentionally self-sabotage later.

Why Obesity and Disease Are So Prevalent

Since the 1980s, the United States government has made nutritional recommendations in what is commonly known as the "food pyramid." These recommendations are reviewed and updated every five years. Most people think our government has our best interests at heart and that the recommendations contained in the food pyramid are consistent with the best science available and vetted by highly experienced and registered dieticians or other nutrition experts. Turns out, sadly, that's not the case.

Rather than by government scientists and public interest organizations, the process of compiling the food pyramid is driven by vested interests and political action committees that advocate for those interests—most notably, grain and dairy producers. The result: Americans who followed these recommendations ate anywhere from six to eleven servings of bread, cereal, rice, and pasta *per day* and only three to five servings of vegetables.

A similarly misguided recommendation of the early food pyramid was for Americans to eat two to three servings of milk, yogurt, and cheese *per day* and only two to four of fruits. Last, it was recommended that Americans eat "fats and oils" sparingly. The pyramid didn't even distinguish between healthy and unhealthy fats. As a consequence, since the early 1980s obesity has skyrocketed in the United States along with diseases that come along with obesity, among them heart disease and type 2 diabetes. Until recently, type 2 diabetes had been known as "adult-onset" diabetes. The name of the disease had to be changed given that so many children and young people now have it.

For the recovery community, the food pyramid recommendations and the consequences that flow from it are a tsunami. Alcoholics do not eat calories, they drink them, and most alcohols are grain-based. Therefore, alcohol is a carbohydrate that breaks down to glucose when metabolized. Given that comfort foods often go hand in hand with alcoholism, in active addiction almost all calories can come from carbohydrates. That's an overwhelming amount of sugar for your body to handle. Add to this the recommendation to eat fewer servings of foods that contain healthy antioxidants and almost no heart-healthy fats, and the obesity epidemic and prevalence of heart disease and type 2 diabetes aren't surprising.

You can use this information to empower yourself. Government bureaucrats, the agricultural and dairy industries, or any political action committees should not dictate your self-care program. You know your past health and using history, how you are feeling at present, and aspirations for how you want to look and feel in the future. It's time to take personal responsibility for the health of your body, mind, and spirit. It's about integrating recovery into all your affairs, most notably the foods you put into your body.

Alcohol Is Calorie Rich and Nutrient Poor

Alcohol is chock full of calories, unfortunately all of which are empty. Every ounce of alcohol contains approximately 170 calories.[33] The calories in one ounce of alcohol are approximately equal to the calories found in each of the following: a seven-ounce lamb chop, a dozen oysters, a five-ounce baked potato, or a seven-ounce glass of skim milk. But all of these foods except alcohol contain many nutrients. Alcohol contains *no* nutrients and has nine calories per gram. With more calories per gram than protein and carbohydrates, alcohol is calorie rich and nutrient poor.

Many studies suggest that drinking alcohol in moderation is a good thing for various reasons. For example, a glass of red wine daily or every other day can be beneficial for heart health. This book was written for people like me who cannot have just one glass of wine but instead finish the bottle or box (the really cheap wine I used to drink) in one sitting and then look for more. For those of us in recovery, even one sip is toxic. Alcohol also disrupts the normal body functions and causes stress to internal organs—most notably the liver. Alcohol blocks absorption of vitamins in the intestines, inhibits the production of necessary amino acids, and decreases your body's ability to properly absorb critical vitamins including thiamine, pyridoxine, folic acid, vitamins D and E, and pantothenic acid, to name a few.[34]

Because alcohol causes stress to organs, your body responds by producing and releasing stress-related hormones such as cortisol. This slows metabolism, making it difficult for your body to process nutrients. Moreover, alcohol and other drugs increase inflammation. In response to inflammation, the body releases more cortisol. Not only is more released, but in adults, cortisol is released in the area surrounding the belly. The stress on the liver and other organs prompts the body to produce a substantial amount of cortisol. This creates the visceral fat that protrudes out and is commonly known as a "beer belly." All of this diminishes the ability of the body to properly process and digest nutrients.[35] In *Eat to Be Fit,* sports nutritionist Mike Foley writes this about the impact of alcohol on the body:

> Even a small amount of alcohol makes it hard to lose fat. It isn't only that you are adding empty calories to your daily intake; even the moderate use of alcohol can slow your metabolism down for days after consuming it because of the demands on your liver and kidneys to rid your body of this chemical that provides no nutritional value.[36]

How Substances Affect Your Appetite

Alcohol and other drugs affect your appetite in different ways. For example, alcohol suppresses the hypothalamic region that prompts you to eat. Early research on the topic came to the conclusion that alcoholism is a physical disease that manifests as a biochemical imbalance of the brain.[37] Stimulants such as cocaine and amphetamine suppress the brain's appetite-control center. That's why stimulants, most notably caffeine, are often used in weight-loss pills and powders.[38]

If you have ever smoked marijuana, you know you can get the "munchies." Pot disrupts your appetite-control center and prompts cravings. The opposite reaction occurs with heroin and other opiates. Those drugs slow down your appetite centers and interfere with the absorption of nutrients. However, when they eat, those whose drug of choice is opiates tend to overeat sugary foods for many of the same reasons that those whose drug of choice is alcohol do.[39] Different substances may behave differently, but all have *some* impact on appetite.

Nutrient-Dense Foods

It's important to transition to nutrient-dense foods. This refers to the nutritional bang the food delivers per calorie. The best example of the importance of nutrient-dense food choices I have ever read is in *Eating Right to Live Sober:*

> A banana and a piece of fudge, for example, deliver approximately the same calories—but the banana has twice as much protein, less than one-tenth the fat, three times as much iron, ten times as much potassium and niacin, over two hundred times as much vitamin A, seven times as much thiamine, three times as much riboflavin, and fourteen times as much vitamin C. And the fudge contains fifty-four times as much sodium.[40]

As the example above drives home, real food that grew in the earth, in this case a banana, has disproportionately more nutrients per serving size than processed foods, that is, comfort foods, or, as Bill W. described them, the sister foods to alcohol.

When You Eat Matters

There's a slogan used in the different recovery fellowships: "Avoid HALT. Avoid being hungry, angry, lonely, and tired." Notably, the acronym begins with *hungry*. To avoid hunger, you learn to eat at regular intervals and provide your body with necessary nutrients. By eating at certain times of day and being aware of the nutritional content of your meals, you avoid the highs and lows associated with hunger, malnutrition, cravings, and fluctuations in blood sugar. It's also important to focus on what you are eating and at what time. For example, you cannot expect to drink coffee in the evening and/or eat sugary foods and then sleep peacefully through the night. How many evening twelve-step meetings have you attended where the coffee pot is brewing, people are drinking their coffee, and then they share about how they are up all night, unable to sleep? The solution for many is to get a prescription for sleeping pills. The pill masks the problem and, after a while, like all other quick fixes, it stops working.

Is Dairy Okay?

It's okay to have small amounts of dairy products in the Spiritual Adrenaline program. Unlike other programs, I don't have an outright ban on dairy. My recommended foods include Greek yogurt without the added sugar and cottage cheese. However, I do recommend you limit dairy for two reasons. First, a great amount of antibiotics and steroids are fed to the animals to increase milk production. What the cow eats, you eat. Given that you are looking to heal your body after years of contamination by substances, you should avoid imbibing antibiotics, steroids, and God knows what else considering how dairy is processed these days. You can buy organic milk, but it's expensive and should not be drunk in large quantities anyway.

A second reason I recommend limiting dairy products has to do with man's manipulation of the cow's natural diet. Cows evolved to feed off grass and their own milk. These days, farmers are feeding cows wheat, rather than grass, in an effort to increase production. The result of feeding cows wheat is that their milk then contains gluten, which causes difficulty for many people in addiction recovery. For alcoholics, wheat is the primary ingredient in alcohol. Many will develop sensitization to grain, wheat, and gluten as a consequence of their substance abuse. For these people, drinking or eating dairy products can cause diarrhea, nausea, or other symptoms. They may not even realize the problem has to do with the presence of wheat and gluten in dairy products.

One last point: you may be lactose intolerant, which means your body cannot digest dairy products. If this is you, dairy should be entirely avoided. If you are going to eat dairy, make sure to have a food-allergy test, including for gluten.

What Is Grass-Fed Beef?

If you are not a vegetarian and plan to eat beef, I recommend the grass-fed kind. The reason is simple. What cows are fed has a major impact on the nutrient composition of the beef. Cows did not evolve to eat grains, which most are fed today. Here is what science has to say about grass-fed beef over grain-fed beef: grass-fed contains fewer total calories, higher amounts of monounsaturated fat (the good kind), *five* times the omega-3s, and twice as much conjugated linoleic acid (CLA) as grain-fed.[41]

Does It Matter Whether Fish Are Farm Raised or Wild?

Simply by perusing the fish counter you will notice that fresh wild-caught fish are usually more expensive than the farm-raised fish. I used to buy the farm-raised, cheaper version. The fish usually looked alike, and I saved some money. As it turned out, I should have paid a little extra as I would have gotten so much more nutritionally. *Farm-raised* means born and bred in pens submerged in ponds, lakes, or man-made pools. Usually, large numbers of fish are farmed in a concentrated manner. This means large numbers of fish are packed into the pond. How do you feel in an overcrowded room with no oxygen and people pushing? Not very good, I bet. Farm-raised fish are under tremendous stress because their pond, lake, or pool is jam-packed to maximize profits. Unlike farm-raised fish, the wild version are caught the old-fashioned way, in the fish's natural habitat by fishermen.

Studies have shown that farm-raised fish are usually smaller than wild-caught and contain fewer nutrients, for example, omega-3s, than wild-caught.[42] The reason is twofold. First, the farm-raised fish are under tremendous stress because of being so tightly packed. The stress results in the fish being smaller and often decolored. For example, most bright-pink farm-raised salmon are dyed to be pink. They lose much of their natural pigmentation as a result of the stress of being farm raised. The second reason is that wild fish consume smaller fish in the natural order of things. Those smaller fish have consumed even smaller fish or algae growing naturally. Often farms only feed them the algae, skipping the smaller fish. Other farms create a meal by mixing dead smaller fish with fillers. This mix is then fed to the farmed fish. There are worse things to eat than farmed fish, and it's a healthier option than many others. However, if you can afford the wild-caught or can get it on sale, you should go with that option. I look for sales

on wild-caught fish and change markets to get the best deals. When I see a
good deal, I buy in bulk and freeze the fish.

What Inflammation Is and How to Get Rid of It

Inflammation is the body's natural response to toxins. In an effort to remove
toxins, the body increases white blood cell production and the white blood
cells go about the work of attempting to attack and neutralize the toxin.
There are two types of inflammation: short-term or acute, and long-term
or chronic. Alcohol and other drug use cause chronic inflammation of
the liver and kidneys.[43] Diseases such as diabetes cause chronic low-grade
inflammation.[44,45] The good news is that by cutting off the flow of toxins—
that is, for those of us in recovery, alcohol and other drugs—inflammation
can be reduced in a relatively short time. Eating healthy foods also mitigates
inflammation and helps the body repair damage.

Organic vs. Nonorganic Foods

Organic refers to the way farmers grow the plants or raise their animals, free
of all pesticides, antibiotics, and steroids. Organic has a specific definition
and the product must comply to label itself organic. These standards are
set by the United States Department of Agriculture (USDA). Here are the
various types of products under the organic umbrella:

- **100 percent organic** and certified as such means no chemicals,
  pesticides, antibiotics, and/or steroids.
- **Organic** means 95 percent of the ingredients in a multi-ingredient
  product are organic.
- **Made with organic** means at least 70 percent of the ingredients in
  a product are certified as organic.
- **Organic ingredients** means less than 70 percent of the ingredients
  in a product are certified organic.

The word *natural* does not mean the product is organic. Natural means
the product does not contain artificial colors, flavors, or preservatives. It has
nothing to do with the methods, processes, or materials used to produce
the ingredients.

Here are the proven benefits of eating organic foods:
- Studies have confirmed small to moderate increases in the nutrient density of organic food.
- Flavonoids, an important antioxidant, increase substantially in organic food. Omega-3 fatty acids are much higher in grass-fed beef.

The downside to organic foods is the cost. If you have compromised liver, kidney, or pancreas function, I highly recommend you go organic when possible. By eating organic, you'll reduce stress on these organs and permit them to heal. The reason is simple: organic foods contain fewer contaminants such as pesticides and heavy metals. However, the lack of these chemicals permits lots of bacteria to grow and thrive. So if you have Crohn's disease (like I do), other digestive diseases, or damaged organs, be cautious and, if organic products cause you difficulty, switch to the nonorganic version or vary it. For example, one day eat organic, the next day eat nonorganic. If you are eating nonorganic fruits and vegetables, make sure to wash them thoroughly. This will remove surface pesticides and other chemicals so you don't eat them, or at least you reduce the amount that is eaten. Another option is to stay away from strawberries and other fruits that grow in the ground and sit in pesticides and other chemicals in the soil.

What Is Gluten and Should You Care?

Gluten is a combination of two proteins that are commonly found in nuts, seeds, cereals, pasta, baked goods, and grains. The natural purpose of gluten is to act like glue and add a hard texture to these crops. It's the hard texture of gluten that makes digestion difficult. This is nature's way of providing a natural protection so that animals, including birds and humans, don't overeat them out of existence. Many processed foods that are grain based, including alcohol, contain gluten as the binder. After years of abusing foods and beverages containing gluten, you may have developed sensitivity to gluten. This can impact how you think and feel, and you may not even realize gluten is the cause. In later chapters you'll learn about tests to determine whether or not you are allergic to any common food allergens or if you have a sensitivity to gluten.

Hunger vs. Cravings

Hunger and cravings are separate things. Hunger occurs when the body signals the brain that it is in need of nutrients to function. A craving occurs when the brain signals that it wants something pleasurable to be created, that is, dopamine, through an act or other behavior.[46] Studies have shown that the same region of the brain is stimulated by cravings for sugar, caffeine, and carbohydrate-rich foods. All of these foods are chemically similar and/or break down in the body in a manner akin to alcohol and other drugs.[47] Moreover, studies have proven that the body goes through withdrawal when it does not get a substance it has formed an addiction to, such as sugar or caffeine, for example. The similarities between how food, alcohol, and other drugs impact the body are many, and the linkage is critical for those in recovery to understand.

The Macronutrients

There are three macronutrients, or nutrients from which we derive our energy: carbohydrates, protein, and fat. It's impossible to discuss nutrition and modifications to your diet unless these critical terms are clearly defined at the outset, particularly from a recovery-oriented perspective.

Carbohydrates

Carbohydrates are necessary for normal body functions because they provide a source of energy and regulate fat and protein breakdown.[48] Carbohydrates are found in plant-based and dairy foods. Many people in active addiction substitute alcohol for carbohydrates in their diet.[49] There are two types of carbohydrates: complex and simple. Complex carbs are also known as starches. Carbohydrates are the primary source of energy for the body, and they are separated into two major categories: glucose and fructose. (I'll discuss sucrose later.) Carbohydrates not utilized for energy convert to fat, so the number of carbohydrates consumed is important. Additionally, carbohydrates come from natural sources, known as "good" carbs, as well as from refined or processed sources, known as "bad" carbs.

Carbohydrates can be addictive. Here's what happens when we ingest too many:

- When a large number of carbs are consumed, too much insulin is produced.

- The constant excess of insulin eventually leads to insulin insensitivity.
- Serotonin, the naturally produced chemical in the brain responsible for making us feel good, goes into imbalance. The person therefore continues to eat carb-rich food.
- Production of insulin rises with each subsequent carb intake.
- Greater and greater amounts of carbs are consumed with no increase in satisfaction.

Sounds eerily like using alcohol and other drugs, right? You don't need to understand the chemical process or what insulin is at this point. What you need to understand is that there are interconnected relationships among the foods you eat, your body's production of hormones and enzymes, your mood, and your use of substances. We use substances found in our food to disrupt normal body functions, and then our drug of choice to cover up the disruption we just caused. This is a vicious cycle that repeats itself over and over.

Experts have confirmed what many of us intuit: your body does not possess the ability to regulate stress eating. Robert Cywes, MD, PhD, an expert in the area of carbohydrate addiction, writes:

> We eat for the nutritional value of the food, and we eat for the emotional value. The body does not regulate the times when we eat for emotional value. When you're having fun with food, more is always better—and the body doesn't regulate that. You have to have very tight boundaries around how much you eat when you're having fun, and what you eat. Foods such as steak, broccoli, lettuce, tomatoes, chicken, eggs, shrimp, and cheese have nutritional value, but they really don't have any endorphin releasing capacity. Therefore, you eat them until you're full and you're done. Sugars, starches, and carbohydrates become addictive.[50]

Dr. Cywes's conclusion is one of critical importance to anyone seriously interested in addressing substance abuse in the long term. "We have developed an out-of-control relationship with a drug called carbohydrate. We eat sugars and starches not because of their nutritional value, but because of the buzz factor and the high we get from it."[51] Once you learn the basics, it's easy to understand why it is so easy to make impulsive food choices over and over. This knowledge is critical to improving your chances of success in long-term sobriety. Even more than that, being aware of the relationship between food and addiction helps you learn to enjoy being in recovery.

Sugar

Sugar comes in three forms: fructose, glucose, and sucrose. Sucrose is the name for common table sugar and is a combination of both fructose and glucose. For your purposes, let's focus on fructose and glucose. Each behaves differently in the body, and both can be addictive. When you ingest sugars and starches, your blood-sugar level rises. To better transport the blood sugar throughout the body, your pancreas releases insulin. Insulin helps transport blood sugar to your cells. Your brain and other internal organs need a regular supply to function properly. Muscles need glucose to support activity and exercise.

Glucose

As glucose is absorbed into your cells, blood-sugar levels are reduced. Extra glucose is stored in your internal organs, such as the muscles and liver, for later use. Sugar and starches raise blood insulin faster and higher than protein and fats. The greater the fiber content of a meal, the slower insulin rises and the more controlled the process is.

It takes the body about a half-hour to settle down after eating and for blood-sugar levels to stabilize.[52] If your diet contains the proper nutrients for your activity level—including intake of appropriate amounts of sugar proportionate to your activity—blood sugar travels to where it's needed in the body due to an increase in insulin levels, and blood sugar rises and falls in controlled increments. However, when insulin has more blood sugar than needed by your organs and muscles and no place to store it, it then stimulates the production of triglycerides, which convert to fat. Over time, cells that are constantly bombarded by insulin carrying excess glucose become insulin resistant. You actually experience a metamorphosis as your body attempts to protect itself from you! As cells become insulin resistant, cholesterol levels rise, blood pressure rises, triglyceride levels rise, and inflammation gets worse. Eventually, type 2 diabetes results, along with increased risk for other serious illnesses, most notably heart disease.

Fructose

Fructose is twice as sweet as glucose and the sweetest of all naturally occurring carbohydrates. As the name lets on, fructose is found in fruit. When fructose touches taste receptors on the tongue, your brain is prompted to emit opioids and other pleasure-related hormones, such as endorphins, which trigger the release of dopamine.[53] Over time, the brain develops an association between fructose ingestion and the sensation of pleasure. Given the pleasurable association, you of course want more.

As fructose is ingested, it is transported directly to the liver. The liver uses fructose, a carbohydrate, to create fat in a process called lipogenesis. Fat droplets can accumulate over time in liver cells and create a condition known as nonalcoholic fatty liver. Alcohol exacerbates the problem, as it contains large numbers of carbohydrates. The high carbohydrate content of alcohol is converted to fat and is also stored in the liver. One can see immediately the relationship between diet and substance abuse, such as alcoholism, and your overall liver health. But the buildup of fat is only the beginning. Fructose does so much more, and none of it is good. Fructose elevates triglycerides, increases LDL (also known as "bad cholesterol"), promotes the buildup of fat around other internal organs, increases blood pressure, encourages cells to become insulin resistant, promotes development of diabetes, and increases the production of free radicals (compounds that damage cells and DNA and can lead to diseases such as cancer).

Starches

Starches found in carb-rich foods like pasta and bread are complex chains of glucose. In essence, they are sugar.[54] During the digestive process, starches break down to glucose, and the process identified earlier is underway. A Harvard study published in the *American Journal of Clinical Nutrition* found that sugar and other starches, such as pasta, potatoes, and white rice, dramatically increase activity in the pleasure or reward center of the brain. The areas of the brain that experience increased activity after ingesting starch are identical to the areas of the brain that are stimulated by alcohol and other drug use.[55] Similarly, researchers at Princeton have found that starches and sugars stimulate the same areas of the brain as cocaine.[56] These scientific links cannot be ignored.

Protein

Protein represents anywhere from 10 to 20 percent of body mass, depending on age, weight, and overall health. The building blocks composing protein are amino acids that are broken down into two groups: essential and nonessential. Essential amino acids are necessary for body function and assist in the production of nonessential amino acids. Protein increases metabolic rate and helps to reduce appetite.[57] Studies have shown that diets high in protein facilitate weight loss over time.[58] The rule of thumb is that if a food source had a mother (in other words, it's animal-based), it is a complete protein—a protein source containing all essential amino acids. Complete protein sources are poultry, fish, meat, and dairy products. Dark meat contains more fat than white meat does. Incomplete protein sources are grains and vegetables. These complement the complete protein sources, permitting your body to build all the necessary amino acids to promote proper and healthy overall functioning.

Fat

Fats, otherwise known as lipids, have a terrible reputation but are both helpful and necessary to the body's proper functions when ingested in the right amounts. Fats are calorie rich at nine calories per gram. Carbs and protein have only four and alcohol has seven. Fats play a critical role in digestion by serving as the essential element for absorption, transportation, and use of vitamins A, D, E, and K.[59] Fat cells also serve as insulation to maintain proper body temperature and are a source of energy in times of caloric need after depletion of sugar and carbohydrates.

Primary food sources containing fats are from animals. Like protein, if the food source had a mother, it has some amount of fat. Chicken and turkey can be quite lean and contain little fat, while red meat normally contains larger amounts. A second primary source of fat is seeds and nuts, which contain large amounts. Most of us use products such as corn oil, peanut oil, olive oil, and coconut oil almost every day and in many ways. Fats are denser than carbohydrates and sugar and are a better source of long-term energy. There are four different types of fats.

- **Trans Fats:** Trans fats are found in processed food products. This type of fat is known to cause heart disease and other coronary problems since the body has great difficulty breaking down these processed fats. Accordingly, they often accumulate and remain in the arteries causing many diseases.

- **Saturated Fats:** Various foods contain different proportions of saturated and unsaturated fat. Examples of foods containing a high proportion of saturated fat include animal-fat products such as cream, cheese, butter, ghee, suet, tallow, lard, and fatty meats. Certain nonanimal products have a high saturated fat content, including coconut oil, cottonseed oil, palm oil, and chocolate. Many prepared foods like pizza, dairy desserts, bacon, and sausage are high in saturated fat content.

- **Monounsaturated and Polyunsaturated Fats:** Polyunsaturated fats are liquid at room temperature and in the refrigerator. Common sources include sesame and sunflower seeds, corn, and soybeans. Monounsaturated fats are liquid at room temperature but solidify when refrigerated. Common sources are canola, olive, peanut, and avocado oil.

Spiritual Adrenaline Inspiration: **Nancy C., North Carolina**

Nancy C. has more than twenty-five years of sobriety. Her drug of choice was alcohol. In early recovery, Nancy competed in female bodybuilding shows. Although she no longer competes, she's a believer in a body-mind-spirit approach to a twelve-step recovery program. Nancy says,

> For me it's not about recovery from alcohol, it's recovery from a way of thinking. It's emotional and mental sobriety. Alcohol was the symptom. Exercise and nutrition, if executed with a clean motive that has balance and is not an obsession, are very grounding and calming.
>
> I have found that eating foods that don't include refined sugar and certain flour products allows me to have a better sense of well-being, takes away lethargy, and gives me a clear mind. Sugar and flour are a close second to alcohol, so at least for most who have an allergy to alcohol, eating sugar and flour (carb loading) induces a surge of serotonin and can create a druglike

effect. It's easier to focus on the concepts in twelve-step literature with a mind clean of sugar and flour products.

Do exercise and nutrition affect my ability to cope with anxiety, stress, and cravings? Yes. This is mainly because dopamine is released as a result of exercise, which is calming to the brain, naturally, but I have to say that breath work and breathing diaphragmatically along with yoga has proven to be a good foundation before doing any weight-bearing-type exercise.

CHAPTER FOUR

Recovery Hormones, Vitamins, and Minerals

All major body functions are regulated and maintained by vitamins, minerals, and the macronutrients discussed in the previous chapter. You must get the nutrients necessary to create hormones through what you eat and drink. Nutrients then come together through the miracle of nature to permit your body to create the hormones necessary for day-to-day health and your ability to function. No one disputes that the diet of most Americans is deficient in many critical vitamins and minerals. Sadly, even among those who follow the government's food pyramid and other recommended daily allowance lists for nutrients, almost half still fail to meet the recommended daily allowance (RDA).[60]

Given your interest in living optimally and providing your body with nutrients it needs to heal from years of substance abuse, let's take a look at what vitamins and minerals are needed to prompt your endocrine system to create hormones and restore body balance.

How Substance Abuse Depletes Nutrients
The emotional and physical stress caused by substance abuse makes it extremely difficult for your body to properly absorb nutrients[61] and weakens

the immune system and your defenses against disease.[62] When your body is put in stressful situations, the amount of vitamins and minerals required for us to function properly increases. Whatever your substance(s) of choice, nutrients vital to maintaining a healthy body are depleted.

The following list illustrates how substances create a negative impact on the nutrients in your body.

- **Alcohol:**[63] Alcohol use is toxic to cells and tissues. To recover from alcohol abuse requires substantially more nutrients to provide your body with the energy it needs to function and undo the damage caused by alcohol. At the same time, the ethanol and other toxins in alcohol alter your metabolic rate and make absorption of needed nutrients even more difficult.[64] The vitamins most affected are vitamins A, E, and D.[65]

- **Smoking:**[66] There are literally thousands of chemical additives in one cigarette. Many of these additives are addictive. Cigarette smoking has been proven to cause pulmonary oxidative stress, thought to be caused by antioxidant depletion. Antioxidant depletion permits free radicals, or renegade cells, to go unchecked and, in the context of your pulmonary health, leads to greater susceptibility to colds, flu, pneumonia, chronic obstructive pulmonary disease (COPD), and, for some, an increased risk of lung cancer.

- **Opiates:**[67] Opiates reduce appetite.[68] However, when an addict eats, he or she consumes foods high in sugar.[69]

- **Methamphetamines and Cocaine:** It has long been known that stimulants suppress appetite. In 2013, researchers began to study cocaine's impact on fat retention.[70] The small amount of research available concludes that for unknown reasons, cocaine reduces the body's ability to retain fat. Meth users react similarly to those who used cocaine except that the effects of methamphetamine last longer and, in many cases, can be more severe, given that meth users also take in a substantial amount of chemical toxins depending on how the drug was manufactured.

Here's a look at the key nutrients you need not just to survive in your recovery, but to thrive!

Vitamins

A vitamin is an organic compound and vital nutrient that a living being requires to perform critical body functions in limited amounts. There are two types of vitamins: fat-soluble and water-soluble. Fat-soluble vitamins are stored in the body, and megadoses can build up in the body and cause side effects and further damage to organs already stressed by substance abuse. The fat-soluble vitamins are vitamins A, D, E, and K. Water-soluble vitamins, when not needed by the body, are excreted when you go to the bathroom.

Minerals

A mineral is defined as a naturally occurring chemical compound necessary for the performance of a host of important bodily functions in living beings. For example, sodium is needed for proper fluid balance and to permit the billions of cells in the body to communicate. Without magnesium, your body cannot convert amino acids into protein. Calcium is necessary for healthy bones and teeth. Minerals are inorganic and do not contain carbon, like most vitamins do. Critical minerals are vastly reduced by alcohol and drug use.

Real Food vs. Supplements

There are two ways to get nutrients: real food and supplements. Many believe it doesn't matter which of these two sources they get their nutrients from, as long as they get them. This is a myth that is important to debunk. One leading expert put it this way: "[Supplements] can plug nutrition gaps in your diet, but it's short-sighted to think your vitamin or mineral is the ticket to good health—the big power is on the plate, not in a pill."[71]

For millions of years, humans survived perfectly well without the supplements that are relied on so heavily today. Let's face it, if nature hadn't provided for all of our needs, the human species would have died off long ago. There are two major categories of naturally occurring nutrient-providing sources: those that grow out of the ground and those that live above the ground. Almost every fruit, vegetable, nut, seed, and grain contains an abundance of nutrients, not just one. This is true for meat and fish sources as well.

Here are some examples:

- **Apples:** Vitamins A, B1, B2, B3, B6, and B12; biotin; choline; folate; pantothenic acid; vitamins E and K; calcium; potassium; magnesium
- **Sweet Potato:** Vitamins A and B; biotin; beta-carotene; carotenoid; choline; folate; vitamins E and K; calcium; magnesium
- **Almonds:** Vitamin E, biotin, magnesium, phosphorus, fiber, monounsaturated fats, phenols, flavonoids, phenolic acid, polyphenols, tyrosine, protein
- **Sunflower Seeds:** Vitamins B1, B6, and E; folate; copper; manganese; selenium; phosphorus; magnesium
- **Soybeans:** Vitamins B2 and K, fiber, potassium, magnesium, omega-3 fats, iron, protein, phosphorus, manganese, copper, molybdenum
- **Kale:** Vitamins A, C, E, and K; copper; potassium; calcium; phosphorus; iron

Fish and other animals provide almost all of the nutrients that are necessary and are not provided by fruits, vegetables, nuts, seeds, and grains.

- **Salmon:** Vitamins B3, B6, B12, and D; selenium; omega-3 fats; protein; phosphorus; iodine; choline; pantothenic acid; biotin; potassium
- **Turkey:** Vitamins B2, B3, B6, and B12; protein; selenium; phosphorus; choline; pantothenic acid; zinc

How many supplements would you have to buy to get the full spectrum of nutrients found in even one of these real foods? Moreover, your body may not be able to utilize synthetic supplements as effectively as the real thing. By combining naturally occurring food sources, you cover almost all the nutritional needs of your body without incorporating industrially created and expensive processed supplements.

Does the Body Absorb Supplements Effectively?

Studies suggest that the human body does not absorb man-made synthetic versions of vitamins and minerals as effectively as it does nutrients from real food. Some even suggest that the synthetic versions can actually harm our health over the long term. For example, those with liver disease or otherwise compromised liver function already have difficulty breaking down and synthesizing naturally occurring nutrients. This is due to fatty liver, inflammation, and other damage to the liver from long-term substance abuse. For these folks, bombarding the liver with synthetic supplements just adds to the stress and inflammation. One proponent of real food who is popular on the internet is Colin Champ, MD, also known as the "Caveman Doctor."[72] Caveman advocates eating a hunter/gatherer diet rather than following the current governmental recommendation. Caveman reviewed numerous studies and found that in the context of cardiovascular disease, diabetes, and prostate cancer, a patient's health improved when important nutrients including vitamins B, C, and E were ingested through real food but not when they were ingested through supplements.[73] Rather than the supplement-provided nutrients being absorbed by the body, they often pass right through and cause additional organ stress.

Vitamin Interactions

Certain vitamins need other vitamins or minerals to work their magic in your body. If you are taking a supplement with only one, it may not be able to work that magic. A good example is vitamins D and K.

Vitamins D and K are both fat-soluble vitamins. Both are absorbed in the body more efficiently when consumed with fat (the healthy kinds). Vitamin D is found abundantly in fatty fish. Vitamin K is abundant in leafy greens and vegetables. Together, these two vitamins help the body perform calcium metabolism. Experts believe the absence of one makes the calcium metabolic breakdown more difficult and, over the long term, leads to osteoporosis or other illnesses such as heart disease.[74]

The entire debate can be easily avoided by simply incorporating real food into your daily diet. For example, throw some kale together with turkey or chicken and you are totally covered. Nature has already taken care of our needs. We just need to recognize the gift and avail ourselves of it.

Avoid Megadoses

Megadoses of any supplement are both dangerous and often a waste of money. Megadoses of fat-soluble vitamins result in potential damage to your body. Fat-soluble vitamins cannot be excreted by going to the bathroom, so the body is forced to store the excess vitamins it does not need. These megadoses stay in your body, potentially causing further stress, inflammation, and damage to your internal organs. Megadoses of water-soluble vitamins result in the body excreting the excess. The big bucks you paid for those supplements get peed right out. If you eat real food, you need not worry about any of this.

Important Hormones

Hormones are produced by glands, which compose the endocrine system. These glands secrete chemical messengers to communicate with other cells in the body. These chemical messengers are called hormones. Hormones are passed through the blood and arrive at a target organ. The target organ has specialized receptors in each of its cells that react to the specific hormone. A cell without receptors will not react to a hormone.

Think of the endocrine system as a series of transmitters, signals, and receivers, with the receptors being the receivers. If the receptor is constantly receiving transmissions or hormones, over time it will wear out and ultimately stop receiving the hormones into the cells. This is a major reason that it takes more and more of your substance of choice to feel the high. This damage also makes it hard to feel normal even without continuing to abuse substances, as the body has a damaged system for transmitting messages. Studies have, however, shown that as your body regains its health in sobriety, damage to these receptors can be repaired.

Dopamine

This neurotransmitter is responsible for your drive and desire to acquire things that are pleasurable. The brain contains distinct dopamine pathways,[75] each of which has a specific role. Among those pathways is one related to your reward center.

Certain behaviors prompt the creation of dopamine, including sex, eating a good meal, listening to music you enjoy, gambling or other risk-taking behavior, and of course, substance abuse. Substances prompt the brain to release large amounts of dopamine at a quick rate. This floods the brain with dopamine and creates a euphoric feeling, otherwise known as getting high.

Only the hypothalamus and adrenal medulla can create and release dopamine, and over time, if overstimulated, these glands can lose the ability to create dopamine. When your body's ability to produce dopamine is diminished, the dopamine receptors in your brain require more and more to derive pleasure. The vicious cycle can lead to anxiety, depression, and a whole host of other mental and physical conditions. Exercise and nutrition can improve your dopamine levels.

Endorphins

Endorphins are neurotransmitters produced naturally in the brain; they trigger the sensation of pleasure. They are usually produced during times of stress or pain but can also be prompted through exercise and laughter. The brain regulates both the production and release of endorphins, and alcohol and other drugs stimulate the production, and then the overproduction, of endorphins.

Endorphins function similarly in the brain to opiates such as morphine and heroin. When endorphins connect with opioid receptors in the brain, they are broken down quickly by enzymes, then recycled and reused at a later time. Opiates such as morphine and heroin are resistant to these enzymes and continue to reactivate receptors over and over, extending the high and the feelings of euphoria. Over time this leads to dependence, that is, an ever-increasing amount that is necessary to generate the same high. This continuous cycle of increasing use eventually wears down receptors and interferes with the production of hormones. Exercise and diet can improve your endorphin levels.

Serotonin

Another neurotransmitter created by the body, serotonin, unlike dopamine and endorphins, is primarily produced in the gastrointestinal tract. Serotonin is recognized as the neurotransmitter most responsible for maintaining your mood balance. Many functions are affected by serotonin, including your social behavior, appetite, digestion, sleep, memory, and sexual desire. A lack of serotonin can lead to increased anxiety, mood swings, and depression.

As with the other neurotransmitters, exercise and diet can improve your serotonin levels. There are a few more specific nutrients that are referenced later in *Spiritual Adrenaline* and are an important part of the Spiritual Adrenaline program. You need not memorize these terms, but you should get familiar with them and use this section as a reference when needed moving forward.

Other Important Substances
Antioxidants

Antioxidants are chemicals, either natural or synthetic, that can prevent or slow cell damage. In people with a history of substance abuse, antioxidant levels are often substantially depleted. Certain cells in the body lack all the normal components usually contained in the structure of a cell. The missing component is an electron, and the absence of the electron makes the cell unstable. These unstable cells are called free radicals. Left unchecked, these free radicals destabilize the body and cause disease. Antioxidants serve as an electron donor, stabilizing the free radical. Everybody has free radicals in their body, but certain lifestyle choices increase the number. Among the causes of this increase are smoking cigarettes, alcohol consumption, diabetes, and excessive intake of iron, magnesium, copper, and zinc.

Flavonoids

Flavonoids are a group of phytonutrients found in almost all fruits and vegetables. Flavonoids and carotenoids are responsible for the vivid colors in fruits and vegetables. Flavonoids are powerful antioxidants with anti-inflammatory and immune system benefits. Studies link the presence of flavonoids in a diet to a decreased risk of heart disease and other illnesses commonly associated with members of the recovery community.[76]

Free-Form Amino Acids

There are two major categories of amino acids: essential and nonessential. Essential amino acids are those that cannot be produced by the body and must be supplied through diet. Nonessential amino acids are naturally occurring acids that a healthy human body can synthesize for itself. This means that amino acids do not need to be digested. When they are ingested, your body is able to immediately synthesize them into other substances, for example, hormones. Some of the essential amino acids include leucine, tryptophan, and valine. Nonessential amino acids need not be provided through diet; they include alanine, asparagine, and aspartic acid, also known as aspartate.

Branched-Chain Amino Acids

There are three branched-chain amino acids (BCAA): leucine, isoleucine, and valine. The name *branched-chain* reflects the fact that all three have a molecular structure that branches off to one side. BCAAs are important as they assist with muscle growth, enhance muscle endurance, facilitate weight loss, help lower blood sugar,[77] and, according to some studies, may even help lessen complications resulting from certain types of liver disease.[78] With regard to liver disease, testing is in the early stages and the results are preliminary. As your body cannot produce BCAAs, you must obtain them through supplements or diet. Those with alcohol use disorder can be so depleted of these amino acids that brain function slows and causes depression, poor recall, anxiety, stress, anger, and frustration.[79]

GABA

Gamma-aminobutyric acid (GABA) is an amino acid (even though it is often described as a hormone given its characteristics and function) that acts as a neurotransmitter in the central nervous system. GABA inhibits nerve transmission in the brain, calming nervous activity. As a supplement, it is sold and promoted for these neurotransmitter effects as a natural tranquilizer.

Electrolytes

The human body is composed of billions of cells. Each of these cells interacts with others to form a superhighway of cells, tissues, membranes, and fluids. Thousands of times a second, impulses flow throughout the body and prompt the creation of hormones that govern body function. All of this is possible due to electrolytes, substances that produce an electrically conducting solution when dissolved in water.

Spiritual Adrenaline Inspiration: Willa W., Maine

Willa W., a recovering alcoholic, is an avid paddleboarder and spin instructor who lives in Portland, Maine. I asked her how paddleboarding, spinning, and eating right have helped her recovery.

> Exercise and nutrition have directly improved my recovery by not only changing my energy levels and clearing my mind, but also creating an incredible inner power that I can draw from every day, all day long.
>
> Exercising to me is not just about looking good and being toned, it's about feeling completely empowered from the inside out. After years of daily exercise, the gifts are exponential. For me, exercise is how I access my temple. It's my number-one priority first thing in the morning. I strive to be better, faster, stronger, and mostly more alive.
>
> Exercise and nutrition stabilize your emotional state, realigning the neurological balance in your brain to achieve a physical and emotional homeostasis. Exercise and nutrition facilitate a segue for your twelve-step practice to take shape and not only transform you, but completely change you. It's a key component to not only getting sober but staying sober and being happy.
>
> My key advice is to get started exactly where you are. You don't need an expert to show you how to do everything. You need to open the door and show up. Whatever it takes, just walk through the door of that gym. Watch other people working out, ask them for tips, or grab a friend if that helps you. But become willing to do whatever it takes and get your ass moving. Inspire yourself with incredible athletic examples, whether it's on YouTube or in your daily life. Each day, do one thing that is out of your comfort zone. Do not be discouraged, and hang out around people who are working equally as hard, if not harder, at being a better person all around.

CHAPTER FIVE

Recovery Exercise

An important component of long-term relapse prevention is developing tools to help deal with stress, sadness, and other challenges you face in recovery. Just because you have stopped using does not mean you are immune from the unfairness of life and sometimes its tragedies. Twelve-step work will help get you through those times. Inventories, amends, calling your sponsor, and doing service work are all *action* steps and forms of mental exercise that help you refocus your mind when it strays.

A perfect complement to step work is physical exercise, a key relapse-prevention tool that enables you to work through physical stress and anxiety in a positive manner. It has long been recognized that aerobic exercise and weight training can help heal the body from certain diseases prevalent in the recovery community, for example, type 2 diabetes and coronary heart disease.[80] In 2018, two groundbreaking studies, one focusing on strength training (weightlifting) and the other on cardiovascular exercise, both concluded that brain chemistry was altered in a way that prompted the natural production of appropriate amounts of dopamine. Both studies concluded that alcoholics and addicts benefit from exercise irrespective of type, and that exercise can also contribute to reducing the likelihood of relapse.[81] As Nikki Myers, founder of Yoga of Twelve Step Recovery (Y12SR), likes to say, "The issues live in the tissues." Physical exercise is an amends you make to your body for abuse you have put it through in active addiction and to reinforce your commitment to live differently moving forward. At the same time, exercise prompts the brain to manufacture hormones and other chemicals that make you feel better naturally. That's why I recommend that you integrate exercise into your existing twelve-step program.

As a result of the opiate epidemic sweeping the United States and the world, large numbers of former student athletes, injured and then prescribed painkillers, have become addicted. An estimated 20 percent of those aged twelve and older have used prescription drugs for nonmedical reasons at least once in their lifetime. About one in twenty high school seniors (5 percent) reported abusing oxycodone.[82] What percentage of these statistics comprises student athletes is unknown. For former student athletes, exercise was a normal part of their lifestyle prior to injury, the introduction of opiates, and addiction, so the integration of exercise and self-care into a traditional twelve-step program makes complete sense.

Exercise in Early Recovery

It's unrealistic to think about getting proper exercise while in active addiction. Self-care and feeding one's addiction are mutually exclusive things. I never woke up with a major hangover and said to myself, "I can't wait to go jogging." The exact opposite was true. I would pull the sheets back over my head and start beating myself up about what I loser I was, how my life sucked, and what a victim I was of everyone and everything. It took years to break out of this vicious cycle. The sedentary, isolated life of those caught in the web of active addiction just doesn't fit with getting out of bed, engaging with others, and being physically active. In *Drop the Rock—The Ripple Effect: Using Step 10 to Work Steps 6 and 7 Every Day*, author Fred H. writes:

> Addiction is the opposite of presence. Practicing addicts' behavior disconnects them from other people and removes them from the present moment. Their focus is entirely on themselves—what they want, how to get it, and, if they don't feel good, how to feel better as quickly and expeditiously as possible. This self-centeredness ripples out into the world in all directions, harming one person after another.[83]

Researchers in Rhode Island surveyed 105 people recently admitted to inpatient treatment for alcohol dependence about their attitudes and habits regarding exercise.[84] More than half were smokers, and of the smokers, the average number of cigarettes smoked was more than one pack a day. Not surprisingly, the smokers reported substantially less physical activity in active addiction than nonsmokers. At the outset of the study, half the total participants indicated that they were interested in a physical fitness program as part of their recovery, one-quarter indicated a slight interest, and one-quarter showed no interest. Of the 50 percent interested, two common themes resonated: (1) willingness to begin a physical exercise program if they perceived the benefits of exercise as outweighing the cost in terms of dollars, and (2) willingness to begin a program if it was shown that exercise could actually improve their health while in recovery.[85]

These statistics seem reasonable for those just entering recovery. Clearly, physical exercise and addiction are not a natural fit. Getting started with something new forced many of the study participants outside of their comfort zone. The question becomes one of willingness to adopt changes in lifestyle to support their goal of breaking free of reliance on their drug of choice. When I read the study, I thought back to which of those groups I was in when I was in rehab. You may want to think about which of the groups you find yourself in right now. Keep in mind that these individuals were surveyed at the time of admission to rehab.

It will be interesting to see if your opinion and the group you identify with change by the end of this chapter.

Exercise Reduces Cravings

Until recently, there were very few studies that looked at whether moderate exercise could reduce cravings in those with substance use disorders. We now have the benefit of an extensive number of studies, all of which conclude that moderate exercise does in fact reduce cravings in alcoholics and addicts.

A 2013 study involved a systemized review of fourteen previous studies. All fourteen confirmed that cravings were reduced through a period of moderate exercise. The 2013 study sought to ascertain whether alcoholics in a rehab setting exhibited less interest in drinking after fifteen minutes of brisk walking. Twenty alcoholics, all of whom were recently admitted to rehab and who had not drunk in three or more days, participated over the course of twelve weeks. Half walked briskly for fifteen minutes and the other half were allowed to passively lounge around. Each was then shown alcohol-related photos and images and their brain activity was measured.[86]After studying the brain activity of both groups over numerous days, the researchers concluded that the group who had walked briskly for fifteen minutes demonstrated acutely reduced urges and cravings for alcohol. Those in the group that lounged around showed no change. The study authors stated, "We observed promising outcomes in terms of mood improvement, reduced anxiety, and urge reductions over the twelve weeks. . . . These findings complement existing work on the acute benefit of exercise for individuals with addictive behavior."[87]

Other studies that have focused on pot[88] or opiates[89] have had the same results: a reduction in cravings by addicts for their drug of choice. Not only did physical exercise help reduce cravings, but in studies involving those diagnosed with addiction and depression, exercise also helped improve the overall mood of depressed patients.[90] In alcoholics and addicts who identified as suffering from depression, improvements were seen within two to four months of participating in physical exercise as a component of their overall treatment plan.[91]

Exercise Creates a Positive Frame of Mind
All the major addictive substances work by flooding the brain with dopamine. Over time, the amount of dopamine necessary to replicate the previous high becomes more and more until it just stops working. The *dopaminergic reward pathway* is the key to getting and staying hooked on alcohol and other drugs. It makes sense to look to natural, healthy ways to stimulate the production of dopamine and energize your dopaminergic reward pathway to create a pleasurable feeling in a more sustainable way over the long term. Exercise is one way to accomplish that in a healthy and sustainable way.[92] An additional benefit of exercise is that moderate- to high-intensity workouts can improve cognitive functioning, in part due to an increase in dopamine production in the brain.[93] Not only does mood improve, but cognitive functioning and decision-making ability do as well.

Here are the types of exercise and the amount of time recommended to reap positive benefits from moderate physical exercise according to the 2013 study:

Activity	Intensity	Duration	Benefit
Running	Moderate	30 min/ 3 times a week	Increase in motor circuitry; decrease in sympathetic nervous system activity during and after; increase in endorphin output
Swimming	Moderate	40 min/ 3 times a week	Similar to running
Bodybuilding	Resistance and strength training	90 min/ 3 times a week	Improved muscle resistance and strength, and lower cardiac output for effort
Dance	Moderate	90 min/ 2 times a week	Socialization and improvement of motor coordination and attention
Basketball	Moderate	60 min/ 2 times a week	Motor coordination, socialization, and general conditioning
Stretching	Moderate	30 min	Increased range of motion, flexibility, and relaxation

Exercise Reduces Stress

Anxiety, from mild to severe, is an underlying condition that many people in recovery share. For many, substance abuse was their way of trying to deal with anxiety and stress by self-medicating. I am unaware of any specific studies that have determined the percentage of people in recovery who identify as suffering from mild to severe anxiety. However, take a poll at any twelve-step meeting and it's pretty likely that you'll find a large number of those present can relate. Learning to cope with anxiety, tension, and stress without one's drug of choice is of critical importance.

A major study tracked the effectiveness of light, moderate, and intensive exercise on 114 participants, all of whom identified as having had serious trauma in their life, suffering from anxiety- or stress-related tension, and using alcohol heavily within the thirty days immediately preceding the study.[94] The study concluded that those in the group who engaged in vigorous aerobic exercise (Zones 3 or 4) of heart rate for fifty minutes or more a week were the least likely to use alcohol for coping reasons.[95] Those who engaged in moderate-intensity aerobic exercise (Zone 2) for twenty to twenty-nine minutes or more a week also saw benefits, while those who exercised with the lightest aerobic intensity (Zone 1) for three to six minutes a week were more likely to endorse alcohol as a coping mechanism. Both vigorous and moderate aerobic activity, as defined above, were shown to reduce anxiety and stress symptoms.[96]

Another study tracked 187 participants in an intensive outpatient program over a twelve-week period.[97] In addition to their substance abuse issues, all identified as suffering from stress and anxiety. This study tracked exercise by participants at various times and intensities. Participants were not required to do any specific types or amounts of exercise. What each did was left to their own judgment, and the information was self-reported. The study's authors found a direct correlation between those who participated in exercise-related activity and the ability to cope with stress and anxiety in order to stay sober.[98]

What struck me particularly was the conclusion of the study: "Even one bout of exercise can temporarily reduce urges to use."[99] This study is not the only one to reach that conclusion; at least two other credible studies have come to the same conclusion.[100] The reality is that all the research speaks to benefits during exercise or the period immediately thereafter. The participants' urges subsided, but did not disappear. Although these studies focused on alcohol, similar studies have confirmed the same results in those addicted to drugs and smoking (tobacco).[101]

Exercise Helps to Repair Damage

Recent cutting-edge studies are finding that exercise can help repair brain receptors that were overburdened and damaged during the years of using. A 2016 study followed ten people who were given an exercise routine over an eight-week period. The routine combined cardiovascular exercise and weight training. The ten participants walked or jogged on a treadmill three times a week for one hour and then engaged in weight training. The weight training combined weight machines and free weights. A second group of nine people were exposed to health education for the same eight weeks. All of the participants had a PET scan at the outset and conclusion of the study. The results were unequivocal: the ten who exercised regularly had an average increase of 15 percent in the number of dopamine receptors; the eight who did not saw an increase of just 4 percent.[102]

Exercise also appeared to affect other components of the striatum, the part of the brain that releases dopamine. The striatum has different regions, and each is related to different brain and body functions. Among the ten who exercised, the average increase in the number of receptors in the associative region was 16 percent, in the sensorimotor region 16 percent, and in the limbic region 8 percent. (The associative region is the part of the brain that handles complex reasoning and behavior; the sensorimotor region controls the planning, control, and execution of voluntary movements; and the limbic region is responsible for emotions, memories, and learning.) By contrast, those in the group who did not exercise showed increases averaging only 5 percent in the limbic region and 4 percent in both the associative and sensorimotor regions of the striatum. The study focused on methamphetamine, an addictive drug that causes the brain to release a spike of dopamine. However, the results are applicable to large numbers of people in recovery, as many drugs and alcohol mimic the effects of methamphetamine in the brain, though not with as much intensity.

The study shows that the body has an amazing capacity to heal. Brain receptors can recover over time. Just by our abstaining from continuing to take alcohol or other substances, things get better. As inflammation subsides, your organs heal and regain the ability to function, even more so if you incorporate exercise and healthy nutrition into your recovery.

Group Exercise Reduces the Risk of Relapse
Having a workout buddy, participating in group exercise, and/or being part of an "active" community increases the likelihood that you will keep coming back. There is no dispute among fitness professionals that the single most important factor for most people to help them stick to an exercise regimen is having a support system. Exercise partners provide a powerful combination of support, accountability, motivation, and, in some cases, healthy competition. Just the way being involved with your fellowship activities and members increases the chances you will continue to attend

meetings, having an exercise buddy or working out in a group may provide the support you need to stay motivated.

What Group Are You in Now?

In the beginning of this chapter I asked you which group you identified with: the 50 percent who were interested in integrating exercise into their recovery, the 25 percent who might be interested, or the 25 percent who were not interested.

Hopefully, if you were on the fence, your attitude has changed or is beginning to change.

Spiritual Adrenaline Inspiration: Sheena A., Colorado

Sheena A. has thirteen years sober. In addition to alcohol, her drug of choice was crack. She cofounded Addict2Athlete with her husband, Rob A.

> Exercise and healthy nutrition increase the chemical releases in the brain that improve mental health and bring about positive mood. I have been able to set new and higher goals to remain focused on sober living through the CrossFit community. The rewards go further by improving my overall confidence and helping me develop a stronger self-pride. Because of the required dedication and this reward system, my stress, anxiety, and cravings are more easily managed.
>
> While twelve-step communities have helped me begin a journey of sobriety, that particular path wasn't a fit for maintaining my recovery. I maintain my focus by giving back through mentorship, coaching, and community building. I personally follow the Buddhist eight-fold path, which includes right understanding, right livelihood, right effort, right thought, right concentration, right action, and right purpose. Exercise and healthy nutrition are simple but disciplined ways I practice and perfect these skills daily.
>
> It can be difficult for women to overcome shame and guilt because of the expectations we put on one another and

ourselves. Trying to sustain recovery with self-destructive thoughts is almost always counterproductive. Forgive yourself and give yourself permission to love yourself again and find pride in all you have survived.

Focus on a healthy lifestyle change, not a diet or short-term "fix." It's important to establish a system of continued goal setting that can leave you a path to continue to follow and grow with.

CHAPTER SIX

Recovery Spirituality

You are about to enter the realm described as a "spiritual kindergarten"[103] by Bill W. in *As Bill Sees It*. The Spiritual Adrenaline approach to spirituality is driven by self-care, learning to love and respect yourself, and the process of putting your needs and desires over those of others. Self-care and the health of your body, mind, and spirit are the foundation of your spiritual program. You should ideally have a healthy body and mind as you work to connect with your Higher Power on a spiritual level. Once you've developed your personal self-care program, you then focus on learning to slow down your mind to avoid impulsiveness and retake control. This teaches you to live in serenity rather than in chaos.

In her book *The Language of Letting Go: Daily Meditations for Codependents,* Melody Beattie defines self-care as "not, as some may think, a spin-off of the 'me generation.' It isn't self-indulgence. It isn't selfishness. . . . Self-care means learning to love the person we're responsible for taking care of—ourselves."[104] Without loving ourselves, it's not possible to love and care for others within appropriate boundaries.

Hungry, Angry, Lonely, and Tired
Remember HALT, the AA acronym for things to avoid, which stands for hungry, angry, lonely, and tired? When you are any one of these things, it

is much easier for you to get annoyed, act out, or say or do something you later regret. More than that, each puts you at risk for relapse. All of these are states of being that in one manner or another deprive your body and mind of something you require. It's a continuation of the cycle of taking your body, mind, and spirit for granted; it's a type of self-abuse. Your goal is to shift from a lifestyle of self-abuse to a life of self-care.

Hungry

When you are hungry, you deprive your body of the nutrients needed to continue to perform basic life-sustaining functions. The organ most impacted by a lack of nutrition is the brain. The brain requires both water and nutrients, most notably carbohydrates, to function. (Later I will introduce you to medium-chain triglycerides, another energy source for the brain.) Brain function, whether normal, abnormal, or totally messed up, is manifested through behavior. So when you are hungry, your body lacks the nutrients it needs to function and your attitude and demeanor change radically. How do you behave when you are hungry? Do you lack patience with other people? Are you easily agitated? Do you become almost exclusively focused on your own immediate needs, including getting something to eat, drink, and use at any cost? Do you start thinking, *It's all about me* and *I don't care about consequences*? I think most people would agree that their thinking and behavior become radically altered when they are hungry.[105] There is a word for this: "hangry." Hangry means when you are so hungry you become angry. Being hangry interferes with your connection to the world around your well-being.

To avoid hunger and winding up hangry, your self-care goals will be to learn to eat:

- clean food
- nutrient-dense food
- appropriately for the time of day (later I'll introduce you to what eating FAB means)
- at regular intervals

By doing these things, you avoid hunger and the character defects that can sometimes result.

Anger

As anger consumes your mind and thinking, it also obstructs your ability to connect on a spiritual level. Anger takes you out of your true self and can turn you into a walking character defect. When you are angry, ultimately the person you hurt most is yourself. Think about this: how many actions have you taken in anger that you are proud of? Not many, I bet.

Anger is a passing feeling rather than a fact. Acting out on your anger never leads you to a closer spiritual connection, only further from it. How many times have you used at someone who made you mad? When you use alcohol or other drugs at others or your problems, you only hurt yourself.

It is imperative to learn to channel anger into something positive and constructive, something that enhances your ability to feel a spiritual connection to others and the universe around you. Some may say that is not possible, but I believe it is.

For example, China invaded and occupied Tibet, tortured and imprisoned tens of thousands, murdered thousands of Buddhist monks, burned and pillaged Tibet's most sacred shrines, and destroyed revered Dharma scrolls more than two thousand years old. The Dalai Lama was forced to flee Tibet over the Himalayan mountains to avoid being murdered and has lived the majority of his life in exile in Dharamsala, India. You might think he would be angry and hate the Chinese. To the contrary, he prays for them. The Dalai Lama is able to find loving kindness and compassion for them. With his deep knowledge and practice of Buddhist teachings, he has been able to accept reality, as brutal and unfair as it is. Anger at the Chinese does not consume and ultimately destroy him and those who rely on his guidance.

I will share some of the techniques utilized by the Dalai Lama in Chapter Eleven. However, at this point, just realize that it is possible to overcome even the most justified anger or resentments. It's critical to our program of recovery, and life in general, to learn to let all of it go. As hard as it may be, we must. For those with underlying trauma that manifests in substance abuse, hopefully as part of your journey and with the help of qualified professionals you can address the trauma. Carrying anger and resentments is an impediment to connecting spiritually in a fulfilling and useful way.

Loneliness

Lonely is just another way of saying isolated, a major no-no if we are trying to connect spiritually. Loneliness and isolation are not the same things as solitude. Loneliness is feeling dejected by the awareness of being alone. Solitude is choosing to be alone and receiving joy from it. In the book *Just for Today: Daily Meditations for Recovering Addicts* (Revised), loneliness is explained this way:

> There is a difference between being alone and being lonely. Being lonely is a state of the heart, an emptiness that makes us feel sad and sometimes hopeless. Loneliness is not always alleviated when we enter into relationships or surround ourselves with others. Some of us are lonely even in a room full of people."[106]

I have gone on silent meditative retreats where the goal is to learn how to become comfortable in silence and solitude. It's a powerful spiritual tool and a way of forcing your focus inward, without the distraction of outside people, places, and things. Again, quoting from *Just for Today:* "The closer we draw to our Higher Power, the less we need to surround ourselves with others. We begin to find a spirit within us that is our constant companion. . . . We realize we are spiritually connected with something bigger than we are."[107] Hopefully you will learn to enjoy solitude as a spiritual tool.

As humans, we are all social creatures; we need to interact with others. It's a basic trait that makes us human. It is contrary to your genetics and best interests to be isolated and alone. Your disease feeds off loneliness and gives addiction power. Bill W. noted: "Without exception, alcoholics are tortured by loneliness. . . . Even before our drinking got bad and people began to cut us off, nearly all of us suffered the feeling that we didn't quite belong."[108]

When you are isolated and alone, the crazy ideas your disease puts in your head may not seem so crazy. How many times have you shared at a meeting about some thought that has been playing over and over in your head? When you share out loud, you realize just how ridiculous it truly is. When you run it by a sponsor or at fellowship, it becomes crystal-clear that whatever your disease was telling you is against your best interests and judgment.

Groups can also act as a support network and a sounding board. Other members of the group often help you come up with specific ideas for improving a difficult situation or life challenge, holding you accountable along the way. Regularly talking and listening to others helps you put your own problems in perspective.

Many people experience mental health difficulties, but few speak openly about them to people they don't know well. Often, you may feel like you are the only one struggling, but I assure you, you're not. It can be a relief to hear others discuss what they're going through and realize you're not alone.

Loneliness and isolation disconnect you from your peers, feed your "stinking" thinking, contribute to a lack of self-esteem, and permit your disease to control your mind and body. When you feel connected to a larger group, loneliness disappears and the collective best interests of the group contribute to a sense of spirituality. When you attend a twelve-step meeting, you share a collective spiritual experience with others. You tear down the walls that you erect to separate you from others and instead come together to share about your innermost feelings.

When you first get to a meeting, do you automatically feel a part of the group? The answer is probably no. After the meeting, having heard members' shares, related to others, and participated in a collective experience, do you usually feel different? Personally, I never left a meeting in a worse place than when I arrived.

The same is true for group exercise at the gym, in a yoga class, or when you participate in sports or other team-based activities. To avoid loneliness and isolation, I suggest developing a self-care program that

- forces you out of your comfort zone;
- encourages interaction with like-minded peers; and
- establishes a schedule of activities at which your absence would be noticeable, for example, a service commitment at a meeting.

Tired

Everyone can relate to being tired. We are all pushed in too many directions, and a typical day can be exhausting. Most people do not get adequate sleep. When you fail to get enough sleep, almost everything seems to change. Researchers have studied the effects of sleep deprivation, and the results are important to understand. Sleep deprivation impairs your judgment, damages internal organs, prompts weight gain, and causes disease and depression.[109]

Think about how you feel when you are not sleeping well or at all. When I was using, I would sometimes stay up for days a time, completely sleep deprived and high on drugs and alcohol. My perception of reality was completely distorted.

A challenge of early recovery is to relearn basics such as how to sleep naturally and soundly. Given that you have disrupted your sleeping pattern for years or had no positive habits for when you went to sleep and when you woke up, all of this can seem relatively new. Those times when I have come close to relapse have one common theme: I was exhausted! I was not sleeping well, and my disease kept telling me that one shot of Jack Daniel's would help me fall, and stay, asleep. Thankfully, I was smart enough to know that there is no such thing as "one shot" or "one snort" or "one anything" and that if I followed my flawed logic, it would turn into a multiple-day bender. Self-care tips for sleep include:

- Eat to make it easier to sleep. (I'll teach you to eat FAB in Chapter Eight.)
- Slow down your brain function prior to going to bed.
- Schedule your exercise to enhance your sleep.
- Manage technology to promote sleep and recognize that we can become addicted to our smartphone, other devices, and social media.

HALT and Spirituality

What does being hungry, angry, lonely, or tired have to do with spirituality? Everything! Each of these is an altered state resulting from a weakness in your self-care. Without a self-care program to avoid these and other altered states, your body is put under constant stress and you continue to cause inflammation and other internal chaos.

Living in chaos is itself addictive. It's a learned behavior that accentuates the effect of alcohol and other drugs. Chaos, as with your substances of choice, becomes a higher power. All of this is fed by technology, which is also addictive. If you wish to attain serenity and achieve a spiritual connection, you must learn to slow your mind down, eliminate chaos as much as you can, and control impulsive thinking.

After even a few days of slowing down and focusing on your higher power, you probably will notice differences—some subtle, some more profound—not so much in the world around you, but in your perception of

it. Journal about these changes, enjoy them, breathe deeply, and recommit
to continuing the process you have just begun.

Hopefully in the next seven, thirty, and ninety days and beyond, you will
continue to grow and change in ways you have only dreamed of while using.
Make sure you recognize your accomplishments as you move forward. Also,
if you wind up not making the progress you would like, you can rework
your program and try something different. Human nature confirms that
many people engage in self-sabotage in a subconscious effort to undercut
their efforts. I can tell you that I am almost always my own worst enemy.
Buddhist monk Lama Tsultrim Yeshe, who teaches overcoming trauma with
Buddhist tools, explains how trauma is embedded in our habits. Trauma
manifests through negative behaviors that become habits, such as self-
loathing and self-sabotage. Lama Tsultrim teaches that by addressing the
underlying trauma, we empower ourselves to break the consequence of the
trauma that manifests as habit.

Rumination is when you get exhausted repeating the same thing over
and over in your head, wishing you had done or said something differently,
or just beating yourself up for being "less than." This is a cycle of distorted
and self-destructive thinking that thrives in active addiction. It's a learned
behavior and something you should strive to disempower. Rumination
engages the critical parent in your brain. The term *critical parent* is
interchangeable with *your addiction*. I think most people know what I am
talking about: it's that nagging voice in your head that tells you that you
are not smart enough, handsome enough, tall enough, fast enough, thin
enough, pretty enough, and that you are basically a loser with absolutely no
hope of ever accomplishing anything in your life.

Almost every morning when I wake up, I hear my critical parent. I used
to listen to the constant putdowns and give those negative thoughts great
weight. After a while, I actually believed them. Recovery has taught me
to ignore self-loathing, although this type of thinking refuses to go away
completely. Immediately after waking up, I read my morning meditations,

take a hot bath, breathe deeply, and then go to the gym before work. By the time I've finished with my routine, the critical parent is no longer telling me how terrible I am. Instead, positive self-affirmations begin to dominate my thinking. I focus on my gratitude for having woken up sober and look forward to embracing whatever challenges I will face that day.

Spiritual Adrenaline Inspiration: Holly F., New York

Holly F. is recovering from an eating disorder. Although Holly did not have a concurrent substance abuse problem, more than 57 percent of women in recovery from substance abuse also have an eating disorder. I asked her to share her experience, strength, and hope with us.

Here is how Holly describes the impact of yoga.

> Exercise was a key player in my recovery from disordered eating. At the age of twenty-two, during the peak of my illness, I became severely regimented about my daily running routine. I would wake up at 6:00 a.m. and run up to eight miles a day in combination with restricting my food intake in order to maintain a low body weight. Eventually these daily habits became impossible to maintain, causing a profound depression to set in. Once I was in therapy I became aware of the fact that I had deep-rooted anxiety issues.
>
> After a few months, with the positive support of my therapist, I built up the courage to try yoga, as I had heard it was an effective way to deal with stress. I found a small local studio in Brooklyn and began taking a beginner's class that met once a week. I remember feeling incredibly uncomfortable and self-conscious during the first few months of that class. But I began to notice that when I would leave the studio I would feel better than when I had walked in. This is what kept me going back.
>
> I had spent years trying to run away from my body and emotions, and I found that simply breathing in the different yoga postures created a welcoming space for me to be present

with myself. I had always felt ashamed of my emotional needs and of the shape and appearance of my body. Learning yoga gave me a new lens through which to see myself that focused more on my inside than on my outside. I took that beginners' class for about two years while also going to weekly therapy. My confidence slowly started to grow, and I also built up the strength to try new foods even *enjoy* a big meal without wanting to punish myself afterward. Practicing yoga as part of my recovery didn't cure my eating disorder. What it did do at that crucial time was enable me to accept myself—my emotions, needs, strengths, and weakness—in a fuller way than I ever had before.

Practicing yoga and meditation on a regular basis helps me to be more conscious of my thought patterns, emotions, and triggers, which helps me to manage the anxiety and stress of life. Since I started practicing yoga in 2002, there has been a lot of research showing how the controlled breathing practices of yoga and meditation balance the nervous system and reduce the presence of stress hormones in the bloodstream. I'm not a scientist, but I've noticed that my yoga practice has helped me to slow down enough to both notice and take in the beautiful moments of life when they emerge.

Instead of my life being awash in anxiety, I've learned how to absorb positive events. This isn't to say that I don't feel and experience the stresses, disappointments, and anxieties of life; I do, but I have more resilience. I will probably always have anxiety, as so many of us do, but the tools and strategies I've learned from yoga and meditation have given me alternative and healthier ways to respond to it.

CHAPTER SEVEN

Getting Started

As you start to embark on this self-care program, it would be a good idea to evaluate where you are right here and now and set metrics and goals for the future. After you set your day-one baseline, go about living in a manner that will bring about the change you want to see happen one meal at a time, one rep at a time, one breath at a time, or one day at a time—whatever works for you. Among the metrics that help you establish your baseline are a food allergy test, blood work, and a food and activity inventory.

We all have different goals. For example, some want to look better and may choose to measure their weight, body fat, or waist size. Others may be focused on improving their blood work to feel better and avoid disease. In the Spiritual Adrenaline program, I offer multiple ways to measure your progress so you can pick those that fit your background and goals.

Food Allergies and Sensitization

In the last few years, science has confirmed that people with substance use disorders have a higher degree of allergic responses to some substances. The process of acquiring a hypersensitivity to substances after periods of long-term use is known as "sensitization."[110] Those who are addicted to alcohol and other drugs become hypersensitized not only to their drug of choice, but also to other allergens, including those found in food. Even if you were not born with food or other allergies, your life in active addiction may have created hypersensitivity.[111] I am now hypersensitive to chocolate since I ate so much when I was a kid. Clearly, abstinence from your drug of choice eliminates that allergen from your system, at least while you remain in recovery. Since so much of the Spiritual Adrenaline program involves nutrition and trying new and different foods, it's important to know whether you've become sensitized to other allergens, most notably those found in foods.

A simple food allergy test will tell you if you have acquired hypersensitivity to food allergens. In the United States, standardized definitions and diagnoses of food allergies have been adopted by our government after years of intensive study by the National Institute of Allergy and Infectious Diseases (NIAID).[112] The NIAID definition and guidelines have now been adopted in many countries around the world. They are the gold standard and are followed by all credible professionals and organizations.

A food allergy is defined as an "adverse health effect arising from a specific immune response that occurs reproducibly on exposure to a given food." Food allergies affect a large segment of the population. The NIAID study noted the importance of vigilance since food allergens are found in eggs, milk, peanuts, tree nuts, soy, wheat, shellfish, and fish. All these foods are prevalent in the American diet. For people with substance abuse issues, food allergies should be even more of a concern since alcohol and other commonly abused drugs are known to increase the absorption of food allergens.

Food allergies manifest in any number of ways. Some experience mild nausea, hives, or irritability. Others suffer very severe symptoms including anaphylaxis, a potentially life-threatening form of allergic reaction.

Thankfully, it's relatively easy to manage food allergies in most people through dietary modification and avoidance of the specific allergen. In some people, hypersensitivity may ameliorate or completely go away over time.[113] You have nothing to lose, and potentially everything to gain, by having a simple, low-cost food-allergy test done before implementing the nutritional recommendations of Spiritual Adrenaline.

Gluten Intolerance

Many alcoholics develop sensitivity to foods from which alcohol has been derived without evening knowing it. The component foods that ultimately become alcohol include wheat, corn, yeast, grapes, sugar, fructose, and potatoes. Studies have shown that up to 80 percent of all alcoholics are gluten intolerant.[114] Given this food sensitivity that has developed over time along with the addiction to alcohol, alcoholics in recovery can benefit greatly by removing, at least temporarily, grains and glutens from their diet. Both alcohol and gluten have been proven to affect the brain's cerebellum. The brain is particularly vulnerable to immune-related damage.[115]

Food and Activity Inventory

Fourth and Tenth Step inventories are key components of any twelve-step practice. The function of an inventory is to analyze past behaviors and your interaction with people, places, and things. As part of this process, you evaluate resentments you have been carrying, wrongs you have done, your character defects that have contributed to the creation of the resentments and wrongs, and your overall role in the process. As written in *Alcoholics Anonymous,* otherwise known as the Big Book, the reasons for conducting an inventory include these:

> We turned back to [our inventory], for it held the key to the future. We were prepared to look at it from an entirely different angle. . . . We resolutely looked for our own mistakes. Where had we been selfish, dishonest, self-seeking, and frightened? The inventory was ours, not the other man's. When we saw our faults we listed them. We placed them before us in black and white. We admitted our wrongs honestly and were willing to set these matters straight.[116]

The message is as powerful today as it was then. In the context of Spiritual Adrenaline, you can benefit by focusing your inventory on the damage you've done to your body, mind, and spirit. You cannot blame others for the food you eat or the fact that you chose to isolate, live like a couch potato, and harbor negative attitudes toward everything. Your poor self-care choices got you there, and your positive choices will get you out. As always, it is your choice and your actions that determine both your present and your future.

Suggested Internal Measure

An important part of Spiritual Adrenaline is taking personal responsibility for your own health. That is the key to any self-care program and a living amends. You cannot take responsibility for your health if you cannot decipher what your blood is telling you. Too often these days medical professionals are overwhelmed and their offices understaffed. They simply do not have the time to review all the test results that come back and effectively communicate the story your blood is telling.

That's why it's important to decipher the most important medical terms contained in your blood tests. You are then empowered to ask the right questions of your healthcare professional and avoid something important being overlooked given the reality of medical care today. The best way to measure your internal health as you start and during this process is through a complete blood count (CBC). This relatively inexpensive test should be performed every six months for at least the first two years of your recovery. "Why?" you may ask. As Dr. Michael Bedecs told me when I was getting started, it's simple: "Blood does not lie." Blood and its components are the best possible measure of internal health and predictor of the potential for future disease or illness. Also, ask your medical provider to use a patient-friendly lab that uses common language or well-recognized symbols. I recommend Access Medical Laboratories. Access provides easy-to-read blood test results and prints your prior test results next to your current results. Access provides up to eight blood tests on one page so it is easy to see how your blood work is changing over time.

Here are the categories recommended for you to monitor. If there is no abbreviation, it's because there is no commonly accepted abbreviation or the full name is used. Abbreviation definitions are provided at the end of this section.

- **WBC** (white blood cell count): Healthy range 4.3 to 10.800 cmm. Elevated levels can indicate an infection or inflammation in organs.
- **Sodium:** Healthy range 135 to 145 mEq/L. An important electrolyte for breathing, nerve impulses, muscle contractions, and other critical body functions. Elevated levels can lead to heart disease and/or indicate liver or kidney problems.
- **GLU** (blood sugar): Healthy range 70 to 99 mg/dL. To properly test your blood glucose, you must fast for six to twelve hours prior

to testing. Given that a disproportionate percentage of the recovery community is either hypoglycemic or diabetic, elevated levels need to be addressed. Blood glucose is directly affected by your diet.

- **HDL** ("good" cholesterol): Generally accepted range: above 60 mg/dL is considered optimal. Between 50 and 60 mg/dL is considered good. Below 40 mg/dL for men and 50 mg for women is considered poor. Known as good cholesterol because it carries cholesterol away from the arteries to the liver where it is removed from the body.

- **LDL** ("bad" cholesterol): Below 100 mg/dL is considered optimal. Between 100 and 129 mg/dL is considered very good. Between 130 and 159 mg/dL is considered elevated. Between 160 and 189 mg/dL is considered high. Above 189 is considered very high. Known as bad cholesterol because it remains in the bloodstream and over time can clog arteries.

- **Triglycerides** (TRI): Triglycerides are produced by the body and are the basic building blocks for fat. Unused triglycerides are stored in fat cells, and over time and based upon diet, your levels may be too high. A high triglyceride count is an early warning sign for heart disease. Normal: less than 150 mg/dL. Elevated: 150 to 199 mg/dL. High: 200 to 499 mg/dL. Very high: 500 mg or above.

- **Cortisol:** Normal range is between 6 and 23 mcg/dL. This level is the normal range during early morning, as levels fluctuate throughout the day. Cortisol is the basic hormone secreted when our fight-or-flight instincts kick in. It is secreted when we are stressed and/or suffering from anxiety. When the body releases cortisol, our digestive system is suppressed and our immune system responds. Cortisol levels also affect the breakdown of proteins, fats, and carbohydrates.

- **Kidney Function:** BUN (blood urea nitrogen): 10 to 20 mg/dL. An important measure of kidney and liver functions. Elevated levels can indicate issues with the kidneys. Medications and a high-protein diet can also elevate BUN levels.

- **BUN/Creatinine Ratio:** 10.1 to 20.1. This is another important measure of kidney function. It helps assess whether the kidneys are excreting waste properly.

- **Creatinine Serum:** 0.5 to 1.1 mg/dL (women) and 0.6 to 1.2 mg/dL (men). Manufactured in the liver, creatinine serves as a source of energy for the muscles. Ultimately, it becomes a waste product excreted by the kidneys. Elevation can indicate issues with kidney function or health.

- **Liver and Kidney Function** (ALT): Healthy range 8 to 37 IU/L. ALT stands for alanine aminotransferase. This is a liver enzyme. Levels beyond 37 raise concerns regarding liver disease and need to be addressed by your doctor.
- **AST:** Healthy range 10 to 34 IU/L. An important enzyme found in the heart and liver. Elevated levels may indicate damage to these organs.
- **Albumin:** Healthy range 3.9 to 5.0 g/dl. A protein made by the liver; levels out of the normal range can be an indicator of liver or kidney disease.
- **Alkaline Phosphatase:** Healthy range 44 to 147 IU/L. An enzyme involved in liver function and bone growth. Elevated levels may indicate liver or bone-related disease.
- **Bilirubin:** Healthy range 0.1 to 1.9 mg/dL. An important enzyme relating to liver and kidney function. Levels outside the normal range may indicate problems with these organs.
- **C-Reactive Protein (CRP):** A liver enzyme that is produced in response to inflammation. A high level in your blood can mean inflammation in the body. Some medical professionals believe the CRP test is more reliable than LDL cholesterol for determining risk of heart disease. CRP is not usually included in a CBC, so your medical professional will need to order it for you. A level lower than 1.0 mg is considered excellent, between 1.0 mg and 3.0 mg is considered average, and above 3.0 is considered high risk.

The Various Blood "Panels"

Here are the common "panels" you can request depending on your health history and goals.

- **The Lipid Panel:** Lipids, including triglycerides, HDL cholesterol, and LDL cholesterol, are fatty substances found in the blood.
- **The Basic Metabolic Panel:** Tests for blood sugar (glucose) levels, electrolyte and fluid balance, kidney health and function, and important minerals and other compounds found in the blood. The

basic metabolic panel is the primary panel to detect diabetes and kidney disease.

- **The Hepatic Function Panel:** The hepatic function panel focuses on the primary indicators of liver function and is used to determine liver damage.
- **Complete Blood Count (CBC):** The most commonly administered blood test. The CBC calculates the different types of blood cells, the number of red blood cells, platelets, white blood cells, concentration of hemoglobin, hematocrit, the average size of red blood cells, and the amount of hemoglobin found in red blood cells.
- **Hormone Panel:** Test to determine correct levels of estrogen, progesterone, free testosterone, total testosterone, DHEA, cortisol, progesterone, and thyroid hormones.

Here is a list of abbreviations that are important to know when deciphering your blood work:

- **Cmm:** Cells per cubic millimeter
- **fL:** Fraction of one-millionth of a liter
- **g/dL:** Grams per deciliter
- **IU/L:** International units per liter
- **Mg/dL:** Milligrams per deciliter
- **mL:** Milliliter
- **Ng/mL:** Nanograms per millimeter
- **pg:** Pictogram (one-trillionth of a gram)

With your blood test results in hand, you can make smart nutritional choices as part of the Spiritual Adrenaline program. With the knowledge you have gained as a result of having your blood tested, and your understanding of the results from a prevention point of view, you can pick the foods that are right for you and customize your program for maximum benefit.

The same is true for your exercise program. If your cortisol levels are high, you may want to focus more on yoga and meditation in the beginning and avoid stimulants like caffeine, nicotine, and sugar. If heart or lung health is your concern, you may want to consult with your doctor and then begin a progressively more challenging cardiovascular program along with heart-healthy foods like healthy fats. If you are looking to add muscle mass and improve bone health, weight training is for you along with healthy fats, lean proteins, and carefully timed carbs. Ultimately, the choice is yours. With the information your blood work provides, you can make an informed decision that is right for your body and your goals.

Before you set your exercise goals, there are two additional blood markers you need to keep in mind. These are growth hormone and testosterone-free levels. Your medical professional will need to order these tests. Each of these has a direct correlation with how fast you can add and maintain muscle, how much you can lean out, and how fast your body will recover from exercising, especially weight training. A fifty-year-old doesn't recover the same way that a twenty-year-old does. To set realistic goals for your program, you should know these levels and get feedback from your doctor or other professionals about how these levels affect your training and results, that is, how much muscle can naturally be added if you weight train.

- **Testosterone Free:** Range varies greatly based upon age. Although testosterone serves many important functions, your level will affect how much muscle you can add, your energy levels, and your mood. In men, studies have confirmed that men with low testosterone for their age are more likely to suffer from depression than those with levels in the normal range.[117]
  - Here are the normal ranges for free testosterone according to age.
    5.05 to 19.8 ng/dL for men 25 to 29
    4.86 to 19.0 ng/dL for men 30 to 34
    4.65 to 18.1 ng/dL for men 35 to 39
    4.46 to 17.1 ng/dL for men 40 to 44
    4.28 to 16.4 ng/dL for men 45 to 49
    4.06 to 15.6 ng/dL for men 50 to 54
    3.87 to 14.7 ng/dL for men 55 to 59
    3.67 to 13.0 ng/dL for men 60 to 64
    3.47 to 13.0 ng/dL for men 65 to 69
    3.28 to 12.2 ng.dL for men 70 to 74
    Beyond age seventy-five in men, there are no normal ranges that are recognized.
    For women, below 1.5 pg/mL for those under age fifty and below 1.0 pg/mL for those over age fifty are considered low.

There are no normal ranges that are well recognized for women as there are for men.

- **Growth Hormone (IGF):** Range varies greatly based upon age. Growth hormone plays a major role in regulating body composition, muscle and bone growth, sugar and fat metabolism, and cardiac function. It also enables your body to heal after injury or vigorous workouts. If you are contemplating a strenuous workout regimen, you should definitely check your IGF. This way, you set realistic training goals and avoid injury by working out in an age- and health-appropriate manner.

IGF Ranges		
	Men	**Women**
18 to 22 years old	91–442 ng/ml	85–370 ng/ml
26 to 30 years old	60–328 ng/ml	66–303 ng/ml
36 to 40 years old	48–292 ng/ml	54–258 ng/ml
45 to 50 years old	40–259 ng/ml	44–227 ng/ml
55 to 60 years old	34–232 ng/ml	37–208 ng/ml
65 to 70 years old	32–209 ng/ml	34–194 ng/ml
75 to 80 years old	33–192 ng/ml	34–182 ng/ml

After reviewing your initial blood work with a trusted medical professional, you should set goals for achieving improvement in important markers in your blood work. This is subjective for each person based upon the individual results you get and the recommendations of your doctor. The major categories and goals you may want to focus on are:

- Reducing your blood sugar
- Reducing your white blood cell count
- Lowering your cortisol level
- Lowering your triglycerides
- Lowering your bad and increasing your good cholesterol

Speak to your doctor about what changes can be realistically achieved over the course of this program and then at six months, a year, and beyond. Only you and your doctor can set those goals in a safe manner. If you do not have blood work done at the outset, you'll regret it later. It's impossible to accurately measure progress later, as your day-one blood work cannot be recreated or even estimated.

Medication and Nutrient Depletion

The nutrient-depletion effect of prescription drugs is well known.[118] Many of the major medical conditions common in the recovery community have medications prescribed as part of treatment. For example, commonly prescribed medications for anxiety, depression, diabetes, heart-related illness, fatty liver, cirrhosis of the liver, and kidney disease all impact nutrient absorption and retention.[119] Obviously, these medications can be life saving and absolutely necessary. I am not suggesting you discontinue your medication; however, part of self-care is educating yourself on your body and its needs. Make sure to ask your doctor, nutritionist, or other trusted healthcare professional about how the medications you are taking can impact your health.

Suggested External Measures

It's time to set future goals and your external measures.

Photos

It is highly recommended you take a photograph of yourself on day one. Make sure you take the photograph with a solid background and with adequate lighting. The reason is simple: you want to continue taking photographs as you progress, and they must be taken in the same location and same lighting to be accurate. We have all seen the infomercials on TV with "before" and "after" photos taken in completely different places and lighting. Of course the "after" photo is shot with great lighting, impeccable hair, and lots of makeup. In stark contrast, the "before" photo is shot in bad lighting, with one eye partially closed and messy hair. I am exaggerating, of course, but you know what I am talking about. You want your comparison to be as real as possible. Being honest with yourself about where you start is critical to long-term success. It will also carry over to other aspects of your life and really help move you in the right direction toward becoming the person you were born to be.

Muscle Measurements

Measure your waist, chest, biceps, triceps, and quadriceps. It's easy, and you can do it all on your own at home. What you will need is a tape measure designed to measure different muscle groups on your body. I recommend any tape measure with a self-locking mechanism. The self-locking mechanism eliminates the need to have someone available to help you. This permits you to measure on your own until you get comfortable having someone else assist. Various sporting goods stores and websites carry these types of tape measures—the less expensive, the better. For guidance on how to correctly measure your muscles, visit www.bodybuilding.com. What I like about this website is that it contains a lot of free, practical advice for beginners, for intermediates, and for those who have been working out for some time. You can also check out videos on YouTube. Just be skeptical and try to make sure the person who posted the video knows what he or she is talking about!

Weight

If you don't have one, it's time to invest in an accurate scale for purposes of checking your weight on a weekly basis. Look for a scale that allows you to measure both your weight and body fat. Although many scales are not 100 percent accurate, they are close enough and will give you a metric or measurement to work with. You do not need an expensive scale that is very accurate unless you are competing and in hard-core training. If your gym has an accurate scale, you are ahead of the game and can save some money. Remember to take your weight measurements in the morning when you wake up prior to drinking any fluids. The reason you measure in the morning is that you want an accurate measurement before eating and hydrating.

Body Fat

If you plan to measure body fat, be aware that measuring body fat on a scale is not optimal, but for beginners it's fine. The reason it's not optimal is that there are variables that cause the measurements to fluctuate greatly, such as time of day and how hydrated you are. Other factors come into play as well because the body-fat measurement is based upon the amount of time it takes a current of electricity to traverse your body.

If you have a trainer at your gym, he or she may have a caliper, which is a more accurate measure of body fat. It is extremely challenging to measure your own body-fat percentage using a caliper. You will need someone who knows how to use one. Inexpensive models can be purchased online or at local sporting goods stores. Although I do not recommend buying the cheaper versions, it might be worth it if you have a partner who can help you use it on a regular basis so the measurements will be more accurate. Usually, if the same person is using the same device, there will be some consistency over time with the measurements. They may be equally wrong or equally right. The point is that the same person using the same device over time will enhance consistency. There are plenty of apps you can download to assist you in measuring your body fat, showing exactly where on the body to take the measurements. Men and women measure in different places due to our different anatomies and body types.

The optimal and most accurate way to measure your body fat is in a "body pod." You can search to locate gyms or colleges in your area that have body pods. The body pod is a small tub you climb into and in which you sit down. It's filled with water and measures body fat by the amount of water displaced while considering weight and other factors. I usually get measured in a body pod when I am about to compete in a men's physique show or when I believe I have achieved a training milestone. Body pods are expensive and cost about one hundred dollars per measurement, so it's not practical to get measured regularly.

BMI Is Not Accurate

You probably have heard a lot about the Body Mass Index, or BMI. It was devised by a Belgian, Lambert Adolphe Jacques Quetelet, in the early nineteenth century. A mathematician, he produced the formula to give a quick and easy way to measure the degree of obesity of the general population in order to assist the government in allocating resources. In other words, it's a 200-year-old formula that is contrary to today's science. It makes no allowance for the relative proportions of bone, muscle, and fat in the body. Bone is denser than muscle and twice as dense as fat, so a person with strong bones, good muscle tone, and low fat will have a high BMI.

Athletes and fit, health-conscious movie stars who work out a lot tend to find themselves classified as overweight or even obese. By way of example, even when I am at 5 to 8 percent body fat and ultralean, I am considered obese if I use BMI. This is due to my muscle mass, which the BMI scale fails to consider. Don't self-sabotage; forget about your BMI measurement.

In July 2018, the Sydney *Morning Herald,* one of Australia's largest newspapers, interviewed five well-recognized experts and asked those experts to opine on whether BMI was a good indicator of a healthy weight.[120] All five stated that it was not. Among the reasons given were that BMI cannot differentiate between muscle and fat mass; cannot differentiate between where muscle or fat is on the body (for example, visceral fat around the belly versus fat on arms or legs); and does not take into account differences in ethnic background, which can impact appropriate fat-to-muscle ratios.

Realistic Goals

It is important that the goals you set early on be reasonable and achievable. Avoid the pitfalls of rumination and self-sabotage. Set achievable goals, and once you have achieved them, set a new goal. Remember, self-sabotage is behavior that is driven by the dark side of your mind. Your disease does not want to let you go. Your disease wants to hold you back and drag you back down to your bottom. You spent so many years in active addiction hurting yourself. Try something new: be kind to yourself! Appreciate your willingness to change, and set a metric that is realistic and based upon health, age, weight, genetics, and goals.

Positive Reinforcement

What makes Spiritual Adrenaline work is that if you stay committed to the program, you will feel and see the changes happen to your body, mind, and spirit. The motivation to continue comes from positive reinforcement as a consequence of healthy living. The compliments people give you, your family noticing changes for the better, and your employer entrusting you with more responsibility are examples of recovery-focused living. Don't look at eating right and exercise as work. Embrace them as joyful things to do and a lifestyle that places your health and happiness ahead of all other things.

More of My Story

I was *not* a believer when I had my first blood drawn in January of 2012. Dr. Michael Bedecs convinced me to try it, and I did so reluctantly. When Dr. Bedecs gave me the results, I was floored. My blood sugar was elevated; I had a five times increased risk of heart disease; my cortisol levels and white blood cell count were elevated; and my testosterone levels were extremely low. Although genetics plays a role to some extent, it is indisputable that lifestyle also plays a major role. Across the board, my blood-test results told the story of how I had lived as an alcoholic and addict, even if it was no longer obvious on the surface. I was shocked into understanding that my lifestyle was slowly killing me. My blood made it abundantly clear that serious consequences lay ahead without a real commitment on my part to adopting a major lifestyle change.

I embraced the opportunity to make that change and started on a new road to health and wellness. I have continued to have my blood tested every six to nine months since January of 2012. My blood work today tells the story of the unseen, internal improvements as a direct result of living the principles of Spiritual Adrenaline. My blood reflects below-average sugar levels, a decreased risk of heart disease, decreased cortisol levels, and an across-the-board improvement in all the important categories measured, such as good and bad cholesterol. Here's a comparison of certain important markers from my blood work over time:

	January 2012	June 2018
White Blood Cell	14.5	9.3
Glucose	118	95
Triglycerides	135	93
LDL Cholesterol	47	69
HDL Cholesterol	48	54

I was forty-four in 2012 and turned fifty in 2018. To see my blood work improve as I age blows me away. If I had continued on the path I was traveling in active addiction, I believe I would by now have developed COPD and have early-stage heart disease and be prediabetic. Instead, I feel and look better than ever. I am excited about living a healthy and happy life. I am even more excited about sharing this gift with you!

To my surprise and delight, Dr. Bedecs described my blood work a couple of years back as being the equivalent of a twenty-year-old Ethiopian marathon runner. Recently, he told me it's more like a twenty-five-year-old Ethiopian marathon runner. Still, I'll take it. This confirmed for me what he told me years ago: "Blood does *not* lie." The blood tests are only the beginning. I actually get excited about going to the doctor these days. I cannot wait to find out my blood pressure, have my lungs tested, and get weighed.

It is a wonderful thing to have blood pressure equal to that of a professional athlete, vastly increased lung capacity, and added muscle mass with less body fat, even as I get older. None of this is unique to me, and you, too, can achieve these results over time by living this program.

Your Food Log

Writing things down is a powerful part of your spiritual practice. Writing with a pen on paper documents the story of you, memorializing your history, permitting you to go back and reflect on your life, and showing the changes taking place in your life as a positive consequence of your recovery.

The discipline of journaling can be a challenge in the beginning. It was for me. When I was getting started with my food log, for example, I would log when I felt like it and leave out things I knew I shouldn't be eating. If I had a half-gallon of ice cream, I would log a quarter.

Over time, and as I started to take an honest look at what was in the log, it bothered me that I was uncomfortable writing down everything I was eating. I started to really think about it and recognized that my reluctance was a form of denial. Why would I put something into my body that I was uncomfortable writing down in my food log? It was as though I wanted to destroy the evidence of my bad habits and I had no problem lying to myself to do it. I started to feel uncomfortable and sad about lying to myself so much.

Slowly, a type of spiritual awakening occurred. I made the decision that I needed to be honest with myself. Not only was I lying to myself, but I also realized that I was poisoning my body.

As I became more disciplined about accurately logging what I was eating, I became more selective. If you are honest with yourself and disciplined about the process, you will likely have the same experience. As your diet changes and you see the results in your appearance and how you feel, logging your food will become a positive thing and help you continue to make progress.

Starting your food log is when you begin to understand the link between what you are *eating* and how you are *feeling*. In the beginning, your food log is simple; you are just jotting down what you eat and when. When I started logging, I used spiral notebooks, a page for each day. As I got more serious about my logs, I stopped using spiral notebooks because I tended to lose them or pages would get torn out. I created a food log note on my iPad. I go absolutely nowhere without my tablet, so it's hard to miss logging what I eat. I often log on the bike at the gym while doing cardio. By using iCloud and syncing my iPad with my home and office computers, I have access at all times to my logs, and in the unlikely event I lose my iPad, I have everything backed up.

Your food log will also help you identify caffeine intake, spikes in sugar, and mood swings. As I began to keep honest and detailed logs, I was able to see late-morning and midafternoon slumps when I was losing energy. For the most part, prior to and after the slump, I was consuming a large dose of caffeine and/or sugar. I started to see a pattern of reliance on these substances for energy, the spike in energy at the time I ate and drank, and then the slump shortly thereafter. You can track how your body feels at different times of the day and after eating different types of food.

Your Exercise Log

Earlier in this chapter, I suggested that you take internal and external measurements. Now it's time to pick which of those works for you and start to keep track. It's best to track your metrics on a weekly basis. Taking measurements on a daily basis is unnecessary and could get you frustrated rather than motivated.

Your Spiritual Journal

Your daily journal is your spiritual journal. It's a daily account of how your twelve-step and Spiritual Adrenaline programs are going. What emotions did you feel? What are your energy levels? What new experiences did you have? What new people did you meet? What are you grateful for? If you've gotten up to the Tenth Step with your sponsor, you can also include your Tenth Step inventory in your journal. "By laying it all out on paper, we give ourselves the chance to sort through what's bothering us. We know we can get to the bottom of our confusion and find out what's really causing our pain when we put pen to paper."[121]

These daily spiritual journals will become among your most valuable spiritual tools. Please invest in yourself, your recovery, and your happiness by finding the time to journal every day. Remember when you were in active addiction and always found the time to pursue alcohol or your other drugs of choice? Put the same kind of passion into getting well and you will see results beyond your wildest dreams. According to Narcotics Anonymous's *Just for Today*, "[T]he rewards we find through the simple action of writing are many. Clarity of thought, keys to locked places inside of us, and the voice of conscience are but a few. Writing helps us be more honest with ourselves. We sit down, quiet our thoughts, and listen to our hearts. What we hear in the stillness are the truths we put down on paper."[122]

Spiritual Adrenaline Inspiration: **Tim M., Florida**

Tim is a recovering heroin addict. To stay in recovery, he integrated CrossFit into his twelve-step practice. After he recognized how CrossFit had helped him stay clean, along with his sponsor and a friend, Tim founded Temperance Training, a CrossFit program, in Boca Raton. Temperance sponsors Sober Sundays, where Tim teaches a CrossFit class to people in recovery. In the summer of 2018, Tim and a team from Temperance Training competed in the CrossFit Games regionals.

> Exercise and nutrition are key components of my daily recovery. I feel that I am at my best when I am exercising daily and eating in a healthy way. This helps me in my recovery because I feel good physically and mentally. This allows me to spend more time reaching out to others who are sick and suffering, and in turn, this helps me.

Since I am competing in CrossFit competitions, nutrition and exercise keep me accountable. This accountability follows over into my twelve-step practice by teaching me discipline in things including praying daily, calling my sponsor, and maintaining regular contact with my sponsees. It has taught me to be patient, too, because you don't see physical results from the gym immediately after a workout.

Exercise is the best antidepressant in the world! I have been there before, unmotivated, sitting on my couch in my own sad thoughts, and just the idea of getting up and getting active seemed like the most daunting task in the world. But, if you can learn to just get up, put some clothes and your shoes on, get outside, and go to the gym or have a bike ride or a swim, the clarity of your mind, body, and soul can turn a bad day into a great day. Same goes when the phenomenon of craving occurs: if I can harvest those relentless using ideas and cravings into a workout or something active, the thought of using disappears and I begin to feel normal again. All of this makes me more motivated and ultimately gets me to work a better twelve-step program.

As the saying goes, "Faith without works is dead." It's about getting comfortable being uncomfortable. If you think that you want to try something and start working out, find your local gym, explain your situation to a coach, and he or she will take care of you. The hardest part is the initial visit. Once you get it over with and start coming back each day, it gets easier and you start looking forward to it.

CHAPTER EIGHT

Recovery Nutrition Tools

Up to this point, my focus has been educational. I've shared basic knowledge about the major components of the Spiritual Adrenaline program. From here on you'll transition to what I call the aspirational portion of the book. You'll put this knowledge to work in your life and integrate nutrition-based tools that can help you succeed. The following are my recommended nutritional tools.

Manage Your Carbs

It's best to maximize the burning of carbohydrates as fuel during the day. That's why I recommend you try to cut off your carbs in the late afternoon, somewhere between 4:00 p.m. and 7:00 p.m. For most people, this will ensure you burn off a good percentage of the carbs you eat before going to bed. By establishing a carb cutoff time in the late afternoon, you avoid putting on fat as you sleep. One last reason a carb cutoff is useful: it will help you sleep. You'll notice that as the day continues past your carb cutoff time, you start to become tired and sometimes even irritable. When you cut carbs off, your brain function slows as the brain and the rest of your body grow tired.

If you start to feel irritable, you can take in a few carbs. An easy way to deal with this is to simply eat an apple. The average apple has fourteen grams of carbs and will get you past that irritability. Another option is to have a teaspoon of medium-chain triglycerides. Coconut oil is a good source of MCTs. This should take the edge off if you are getting irritable.

Remember, the foods you eat send signals to your brain about what you are intending to do. Large, late-night carb intake sends the wrong signal to your brain. Rather than your brain gearing up for sleep, it is gearing up for activity. It's best to avoid confusing your brain by eating the wrong things at the wrong time.

Learn to Time Your Meals

2½ Hours Between Meals

By structuring your meals in three-hour cycles throughout the day, you are burning the macronutrients you take in to avoid excess consumption. I recommend meals two and a half to three hours apart. This maximizes your metabolism and keeps you burning fuel as efficiently as possible all day long. If you follow this recommendation, you should be enjoying six meals a day, or forty-two per week. Three of your daily meals are large in portion and the other three are snacks.

Here is an example of what a typical day looks like.

6:30 a.m.	Breakfast
9:00 a.m.	Morning Snack
11:30 a.m.	Lunch
2:00 p.m.	Afternoon Snack
5:00 p.m.	Dinner
7:30 p.m.	Late-Night Snack

Any excess energy needs will come from your fat stores. When you burn fat for energy and avoid adding new fat stores by binge eating or eating the wrong food at the wrong time of the day, you become leaner. Moreover, timed meals approximately three hours apart will go a long way toward stabilizing your blood sugar throughout the day.

Eat FAB

Remember, you want to eat FAB.

F is for *fuel*. During the morning, you fuel up to get through your day. For most people, that's from 5:00 a.m. to noonish. This is the time of day to eat larger amounts of carbs and healthy fats to provide you with fuel. Make sure to have some lean protein in the morning as well.[123] In her book *Potatoes Not Prozac: Solutions for Sugar Sensitivity,* Kathleen DesMaisons, PhD, recommends that sugar-sensitive people eat protein with breakfast every day, as protein breaks down slowly and creates a steady stream of amino acids in the body, helping to stabilize blood sugar.[124] According to Dr. DesMaisons, "Protein gets tryptophan into your bloodstream. The potato or sweet potato helps carry the tryptophan across the brain barrier and into the brain . . . more tryptophan means more serotonin."[125] Research conducted by groups including the Obesity Society have confirmed the role of protein and healthy fats as part of breakfast to stabilize blood sugar while prompting the production of healthy hormones.[126]

Green vegetables and fruit (within limits, given that fruit, as will be discussed later, contains high levels of fructose) are exceptionally effective for boosting energy in the morning, and they provide a much healthier alternative to caffeine and processed sugar. By slowly incorporating green veggies and fruit into your morning routine, you are teaching your body to use a healthy and efficient source of energy. Spinach, broccoli, peas, and Brussels sprouts pack a potent punch and are great in egg-white omelets to start the day. A half-cup contains the following amounts of protein:

- Spinach = 3 grams
- Broccoli = 2.6 grams
- Peas = 3.5 grams
- Brussels sprouts = 2 grams

All these veggies are packed with the right mix of macronutrients needed to restore your body to optimal function in recovery.

Green veggies, especially spinach, also contain about 20 percent of your RDA for iron. Iron is an essential nutrient and is directly related to energy levels.[127] Iron helps your body create energy in two ways. It is a necessary component in chemical reactions that create energy, and it keeps your blood healthy and able to transmit oxygen throughout the body.

Sweet potatoes are another great way to get energy, because they are packed with complex carbs. The complex carbs will break down slowly over the day, so rather than giving you a quick jolt of energy, sweet potatoes provide sustained energy. When I am in the mood for something different for breakfast, I whip up sweet potato pancakes. This is just one example of a healthy variation on a much-loved comfort food.

Bananas are low in calories and rich in antioxidants and complex carbs. They are perfect to get your morning going, although the energy derived from a banana won't last over the course of your day. The downside to bananas is the amount of sugar. Bananas are among the fruits with the highest amount of sugar.

Citrus fruits should also be a critical part of your morning routine. Citrus fruits are chock-full of vitamin C. Vitamin C plays a key role in helping your body form amino acids that create and regulate energy. A well-known sign of vitamin C deficiency is fatigue. If you combine citrus fruits with the green leafy veggies mentioned earlier, you'll be ahead of the game, as vitamin C enhances the body's ability to absorb iron.[128]

A is for *active*. This refers to the middle of the day when you need to remain active and in motion—for most folks that is noon until about 4:00 p.m. At this point in the day, you start transitioning from carbs to higher amounts of healthy fats and protein. These macronutrients continue to provide sustainable energy without spiking and dropping your blood sugar. They also do not create anxiety and stress you out like large amounts of caffeine. If you are having a stressful day and need more energy, you can consume more proteins, healthy fats, and, if necessary, a moderate amount of carbs. This helps you get through the active part of your day and begins the transition to evening and night.

B is for *build*. In the evening and overnight, you want to maintain muscle and permit the body to repair itself from exercise, stress, or other exertion during the day—for most people that is 5:00 p.m. to bedtime. During this period, increase proteins and greens to permit your body to repair and regenerate as you sleep. Nutrient-dense foods are good for later in the evening before going to bed. These foods require more effort to be broken down in the body and result in an increase in your metabolism.

My "Eat to be FAB" recommendations incorporate the wisdom of the ancients. They are based upon and interrelated with the teachings of traditional Chinese medicine. The human body follows a cycle of cleansing and detoxing. Each of the major organs and body systems has a set time for the natural detox process.

Fuel: 5:00 to 11:00 a.m.

5:00 to 7:00 a.m.	Large Intestines
7:00 to 9:00 a.m.	Stomach
9:00 to 11:00 a.m.	Pancreas/Spleen

Active: 11:00 a.m. to 5:00 p.m.

11:00 a.m. to 1:00 p.m.	Heart
1:00 to 3:00 p.m.	Small Intestine
3:00 to 5:00 p.m.	Kidneys

Build: 5:00 p.m. to 5:00 a.m.

5:00 to 7:00 p.m.	Kidneys
7:00 to 9:00 p.m.	Circulation (nutrients are carried to cells)
9:00 to 11:00 p.m.	Endocrine System
11:00 p.m. to 1:00 a.m.	Gallbladder
1:00 to 3:00 a.m.	Liver
3:00 to 5:00 a.m.	Lungs

Manage Your Sweet Tooth: Sugar Substitutes

None of us are willing to give up our sweet tooth, but because of all the nutritional knowledge we now possess, it's clear you can have your cake and eat it, too! The only caveat: you must change the ingredients in the recipe. Here's how. There are seven major alternatives to processed sugar that I recommend you try in order to bring down blood glucose levels without losing the enjoyment desserts and other sweets offer.

Stevia

Stevia is made from natural sweet leaves and has been used by humans for centuries. It is a well-known component for treating diabetes in many Asian countries. It's a nutritious herb with good iron and fiber content[129] and will not affect your blood-sugar level.[130] For diabetics or hypoglycemics in recovery, stevia is a godsend. Stevia contains no calories, which is helpful in an overall plan to restore balance to your body, and is available in either liquid or powdered form. I recommend the liquid, which is 100 percent natural; just make sure you get the alcohol-free version, which is often made with glycerin. The powdered version usually contains fillers you do not need, such as dextrose or erythritol.

Raw Honey

Honey is a natural, unprocessed form of sugar. Raw honey contains natural antibacterials, boosts the immune system, promotes digestive health, and is high in antioxidants. It's lower on the glycemic index than processed sugar and will help stabilize blood-sugar levels if you use it sparingly. Don't overdo it.

Xylitol

Xylitol is a sugar alcohol used as a sweetener with negligible effects on blood sugar and insulin. It is as sweet as refined sugar but contains 40 percent fewer calories. The "alcohol" in xylitol is not fermented and is not the type of alcohol that is of concern for those with alcohol use disorder. In other words, it will not get you drunk. Xylitol carries a low glycemic load and has a number of other benefits, for example, killing bad bacteria in the mouth and promoting dental health. The major issue of concern is for pet owners. Dogs and cats cannot consume xylitol. It is toxic and can cause serious and potentially fatal illness if ingested.[131]

Swerve

The newest alternative sweetener is Swerve. Swerve can be used for baking or as a sweetener in drinks or food. Swerve is made of erythritol, oligosaccharides, and "natural" flavors. The natural flavors used, according to the company website, come from citrus fruit. Swerve has no calories and is used in equal amounts as refined sugar. In other words, if a recipe recommends one cup of sugar, use one cup of Swerve. According to the website, Swerve does not raise blood sugar or insulin levels. If you have a history of digestive tract issues, you may want to stay away. The reason Swerve has no calories is that the ingredients cannot be broken down by the body and therefore will be excreted when you go to the bathroom. For people like me with Crohn's disease or other digestive disease, my recommendation is to give Swerve a try to see if it "agrees" with you. You have nothing to lose, and all reports on this product to date have been positive. However, given that Swerve is relatively new, I am not aware of any research that has tested the long-term benefits or detriments of using Swerve.

Date Sugar

For baking, I recommend date sugar. Date sugar is made from crushed dates, which are then refined. In most baking recipes, sugar or brown sugar can be replaced with date sugar without a reduction in overall sweetness. When using date sugar to replace brown sugar, use two-thirds of the recommended amount of brown sugar and add one-third of the total amount as date sugar. Date sugar is far sweeter than brown sugar and carries a lower glycemic load.

Tapioca Starch

Another option for baking is tapioca starch. This starch is made from the root of the cassava plant. It's gluten free and has a relatively small amount of protein. It's also low in sugar.

Coconut Flour

A third option for baking is coconut flour. It's high in fiber, protein, and healthy fats. It's gluten free and is also low in sugar.

Artificial Sweeteners

A word is in order regarding artificial sweeteners. These products seem like the easy answer to reducing sugar consumption and the consequences that come along with it. Recently, however, watchdog group Nutrition Action issued a study on the topic called *Sweet Nothings: Safe or Scary? The Inside Scoop on Sugar Substitutes.*[132]

> All have a sweet taste, but the similarity ends there. They have different levels of sweetness, they taste somewhat different from one another and from sugar, they have different chemical structures, the body handles them differently, the amount of testing they've undergone varies, and some are safer than others.

As with most things in life, if a sweetener comes from the earth rather than from a laboratory, it is almost always better for you. I feel it is important to focus on reducing the intake of synthetic or manufactured substances, and if you are going to replace sugar with a substitute, it makes sense to do so with a natural product that has been deemed safe. As so many alcoholics are diabetic or hypoglycemic, it's important to note that artificial and naturally derived sweetener alternatives do not contain carbohydrates, and studies have concluded that they *do not* increase blood-sugar levels. The one exception is saccharin; studies have shown that saccharin raises blood-sugar levels.[133]

Aspartame

Aspartame is an artificial sweetener composed of phenylalanine, aspartic acid, and methanol. Studies show that these chemicals, both individually and collectively, negatively affect neurotransmitter regulation in the brain.[134] Additional studies have linked the use of aspartame to the production of dopamine in the brain. For example, a 2008 study published in the *European Journal of Clinical Nutrition* linked long-term aspartame use to direct and indirect cellular effects on the brain, depression, and other "mental disorders."[135]

Avoid Juicing

I don't recommend juicing, as it removes much of the necessary fiber from fruits and vegetables. Fiber is an important player in regulating blood-sugar levels. With a juice, there is more swallowing than chewing, so naturally occurring sugars are not processed in the way nature intended—broken down in the mouth and slowly absorbed into the bloodstream. Drinking fruit juice provides a massive sugar rush in seconds. It's exactly the vicious cycle we are trying to avoid. Juicing is expensive as well, since it is so trendy right now. By not juicing, not only will you avoid spiking your blood sugar, but you'll also save money. Although I prefer you eat your green veggies to benefit from the fiber, a "green smoothie," made primarily of green veggies, is preferable to a fruit-based smoothie.

Similarly, caution is recommended when purchasing fruit juice at the market. Studies have linked the extremely high sugar content in fruit juice to obesity and diabetes.[136] Given the indisputable evidence that a large number of those with substance use disorders are already prediabetic, diabetic, or hypoglycemic, this is a major issue and should be of great concern.

Instead, *eat the fruit itself* with the skin and fiber. You can also go to a natural food market and look at juice labels to locate a juice you like with a low sugar content, or just water down your normal orange, cranberry, or apple juice to dilute it. I drink orange juice diluted with water almost every morning. I mix a quarter-cup of juice with one cup of water. I also dilute Gatorade, which is high in sugar.

Blood-Sugar-Reducing Spices, Herbs, and Other Flavor Enhancers

Nature provides the most potent blood-sugar-reducing substances. Many studies have confirmed the power of garlic and certain spices and herbs to help stabilize blood sugar. In addition, research has found that a number of these natural alternatives outperform prescription medications for some study participants.

Some people I have worked with have told me that they incorporated the spices into their diet, but don't feel any different. I ask them if they have checked their blood work, and most often they have not. The fact of the matter is that the benefits of these spices will first appear in your blood and later manifest in energy, improved skin tone and color, better digestion, and increased energy, and will naturally lessen stress and anxiety. To maximize your ability to see the changes happening inside you by incorporating these spices into your daily meal plan over a period of three to six months, you must have your day-one blood work done before starting.

Turmeric

Turmeric contains compounds called curcuminoids that have medicinal properties. The most potent is curcumin. Curcumin has powerful anti-inflammatory and antioxidant properties. In studies, patients suffering from depression who were given turmeric over a course of several weeks experienced improvement similar to the results achieved by patients taking Prozac.[137]

Ginger

This root contains powerful medicinal properties as an antioxidant and reduces inflammation. Ginger helps stabilize blood-sugar levels and may help improve early-stage heart disease. In a recent study of forty-one participants with type 2 diabetes, patients ingesting two grams of ginger per day lowered their fasting blood sugar (meaning that the patient had not eaten for twelve hours prior to testing) by 12 percent. In the same study, blood markers indicative of heart disease were reduced by 28 percent.[138]

Cinnamon

Not only is it delicious, but cinnamon also helps to lower blood-sugar levels and has powerful antidiabetic effects. Its medicinal properties are derived from cinnamaldehyde, chromium, and polyphenols. Chromium and polyphenols from cinnamon improve insulin sensitivity.[139] Insulin sensitivity is the term used to describe how sensitive your body is to the effects of insulin. A person who has low insulin sensitivity requires larger amounts of insulin either created in their pancreas or injected in order to maintain blood-sugar levels. If your body is having difficulty metabolizing glucose, you may have what is referred to as "insulin resistance." Cinnamon lowers blood sugar in a number of ways, but mostly by slowing the breakdown of carbs during the digestive process. Tests show that the impact of cinnamon on lowering blood sugar is twenty times higher than that of other spices with medicinal qualities. In studies, participants given a dose of one-half to two teaspoons of cinnamon a day lowered fasting blood sugar by 10 to 29 percent.[140]

Berberine

Berberine is an herb used in ancient China as a broad-spectrum antimicrobial medicine. Over the last few decades, studies have examined the use of berberine for benefits relating to the cardiovascular system and significant anti-inflammatory activity.[141] Berberine has been shown to lower elevated blood glucose as effectively as prescription medication.[142] It is believed berberine assists the body by inducing glycolysis and preventing insulin resistance.[143] Berberine has also been shown to lower total cholesterol, LDL cholesterol, and triglycerides.[144] For those with liver disease, berberine has been shown to alleviate fat buildup in the liver[145] and the causes of fibrosis.[146]

Cumin

Cumin is an excellent source of energy, thiamine, riboflavin, niacin, iron, manganese, copper, calcium, magnesium, phosphorus, potassium, and vitamins A, C, E, and B6. Cumin is also rich in protein, amino acids, dietary fiber, and some fats and fatty acids. Studies have shown that cumin can help people avoid diabetes by helping to stabilize blood sugar. Cumin also has nutritional properties (caffeine and oils) that help those with asthma and bronchitis and may offer some relief from congestion in smokers.

Garlic

(used as a flavor enhancer the way spices and herbs are used)

Garlic's medicinal qualities are derived from allicin, which is highly beneficial to the heart. Studies confirm that it lowers total cholesterol and LDL cholesterol by 10 to 15 percent on average.[147] Garlic contains large amounts of manganese, selenium, fiber, and vitamins B6 and C. Garlic helps strengthen the immune system, contains antioxidants, and lowers bad cholesterol.

Nutmeg

Nutmeg also contains antioxidants and is known to have therapeutic benefits as an antidepressant, aphrodisiac, and digestive health stabilizer. Nutmeg contains a substantial mix of vitamins and minerals, including B-complex vitamins, vitamin C, folic acid, riboflavin, niacin, iron, zinc, and magnesium. Nutmeg has been proven to help boost energy, alleviate symptoms of depression, and stabilize blood sugar. Nutmeg also has detox qualities for the liver, kidneys, and pancreas.

Paprika

Paprika is a great source of thiamine, magnesium, dietary fiber, riboflavin, niacin, iron, potassium, and vitamins A, B6, C, E, and K. This spice packs a nutritional and medicinal punch. Paprika contains carotenoids and antioxidants that help stabilize blood sugar and detox the liver, kidneys, and pancreas.

Vanilla

Vanilla contains substantial antioxidants and has anti-inflammatory properties. Vanilla is also thought to help lower bad cholesterol, stabilize blood sugar, and open airways and provide relief to smokers who are congested or suffering from lung-related illness. Vanilla may have properties that help relieve anxiety. Make sure to use alcohol-free vanilla products, as vanilla extract normally contains substantial amounts of alcohol.

Healthy Late-Night Snacks

Especially early on in the process of change, your brain and body will protest anything other than what it has known, whether it is a good or bad habit.

I used to enjoy late-night snacking and often woke up throughout the night to eat. When I was a child, my father would wake up in the middle of the night and eat an entire pint of ice cream. Just as genetics passes down traits, so does your childhood observation of behaviors of your parents. My father was also an alcoholic. I watched all the negative behaviors associated with his disease and said that would never happen to me. But it did. If you are anything like me, anticipate difficulty late at night when you are trying to go to bed *without* eating snacks immediately before. I recommend your last snack or meal before you go to bed consist of low-carb, filling foods. Following are some good choices.

Rice Cakes

Rice cakes are dense, and one or two will fill your stomach with a minimal caloric and carb intake. A typical rice cake has thirty-five calories with seven grams of carbohydrate. This is tremendous bang for the buck, and if you eat three or four to fill yourself up, you don't need to feel a lot of guilt. If rice cakes are too bland for you, spread some all-natural peanut or almond butter on them.

Ezekiel Bread

Ezekiel bread is based upon a recipe in the Bible. It's primarily made of sprouts rather than grain. If you have gluten sensitivity, "e-bread" is for you. This is also true for diabetics and hypoglycemics. A typical slice of e-bread contains eighty calories, five grams of protein, twelve grams of carbohydrate, and almost no fat. It's delicious and has more complex carbs and other nutrients than wheat or oat breads. It will fill you up, and you won't feel guilty. My favorite e-bread is cinnamon and raisin. You'll find e-bread in the freezer section at your supermarket.

Casein Protein

Casein protein is a type of protein that breaks down slowly in the digestive system. It is usually taken by bodybuilders or others in training to maintain muscle mass overnight as they sleep. However, not just bodybuilders are concerned about preserving muscle mass. Those with osteoporosis or others looking to improve their bone density or overall bone health will find casein protein helpful. It's thick and also helps to make you feel full, which is beneficial late at night when you are getting ready for or already in bed.

Frozen Blueberries

Frozen blueberries are a tasty treat that will fill you up, provide you with antioxidants, and satisfy your sweet tooth. At one calorie each and one-tenth of a gram of carbohydrate, you can have a handful and not worry about the intake of a lot of carbs before bedtime.

Multigrain Pretzels

This snack will fill you up, and since it contains complex carbs, it is a healthier alternative to the standard bleached-flour pretzel. The average multigrain pretzel is eleven calories. To add taste, you can spread an all-natural mustard with no fat, no sugar, and no carbs onto it.

Popcorn

The air-popped version will fill you up and provide you with fiber and a small number of carbs. One cup of air-popped popcorn has thirty-one calories and six grams of carbohydrate. To add some taste, try all-natural flavor enhancers, such as rosemary, Himalayan rock salt, and/or coconut oil, which you can find at natural food markets, and then shake well.

Unsalted Almonds

Like most nuts, these contain a higher fat content than most of the other snacks I recommend. That said, almonds contain the good fat our body needs. Two tablespoons or twenty-eight grams of almonds contain about 180 calories; calories from fat constitute 140. Each serving contains fifteen grams of fat and six grams of carbohydrate. Studies find that people who eat tree nuts such as cashews, almonds, and pistachios, as well as legumes such as peanuts, live longer and healthier lives. They also have less risk of chronic disease, including heart disease, respiratory problems, and type 2 diabetes.[148] Richard Mattes, PhD, of Purdue University, notes that tree nuts are "high in protein, and protein is satisfying; high in fiber, and fiber is satisfying; [and] rich in unsaturated fats. Snacking on nuts makes it likely that you will eat less later in the same day." Following this logic, a handful of nuts prior to going to bed should help you feel full through the night and avoid hunger pangs.

Liquid Egg Whites

Egg whites are incredibly easy to prepare. All you need to do is measure the amount you want and pour it into a skillet. No cracking eggs, no mess, no drama. If you feel the urge, throw in some veggies and create an anytime omelet. When I was struggling to break the bad habit of eating high-fat or sugary snacks late at night, I would prepare egg whites with tomato and onion, and if I got hungry I would eat it late at night or overnight. If I didn't eat it in the evening, I had it for breakfast the next morning. This is a highly practical tool to help fill you up, avoid being hungry, and break the cycle of eating high-fat or high-sugar foods late at night.

Two egg whites will fill you up with about sixty calories, twelve grams of protein, and only three grams of carbohydrate. You really cannot go wrong with an anytime omelet if you stay away from cheese and bacon. If you want cheese, use less, and substitute turkey bacon for pork bacon.

Cottage Cheese

I recommend a low-fat version made with skim milk or 2 percent milk. This is a powerhouse for weight control and/or adding muscle. It will fill you up, and your average five-ounce serving will set you back only eighty calories and five grams of carbohydrate. You can throw in frozen blueberries and a tablespoon of almonds and create a tasty treat with zero guilt.

Manage Your Caffeine

Luckily there are plenty of options for those looking to cut back on caffeine intake. From my own experience, I overindulged with caffeine in an attempt to replicate the rush of cocaine. All it did was keep me extremely anxious and hyper during my initial year of recovery. I had to come to terms with my substitution of caffeine to create a high that was less potent than, but similar in many ways to, cocaine. Moreover, overindulgence in caffeine was the gateway drug to cigarettes for me. One drug enhances the perceived pleasure of the other. It's a vicious cycle. Awareness of caffeine intake is critical in recovery.

Like sugar, caffeine is all over the place. For example, Anacin has thirty-two milligrams of caffeine per tablet. Excedrin Extra Strength contains 130 milligrams per tablet. Popular over-the-counter weight-loss products like Dexatrim and preworkout powders contain large amounts of caffeine.[150] According to the FDA, caffeine is being added to a growing number of products from jellybeans, waffles, bottled water, and potato chips to even gum and candy.[151]

One more important point must be made here: many coffee shops offer caffeine-enhanced coffee. While the average eight-ounce cup of coffee contains anywhere from ninety-five to 200 milligrams of caffeine, Starbucks offers up to 415 milligrams in their twenty-ounce Venti. Not to be outdone, Dunkin' Donuts offers up to 436 milligrams in their twenty-ounce large with a "turbo shot." These are incredible amounts of caffeine in one cup. This doesn't even take into consideration that some coffees at Starbucks and other coffee shops contain as much sugar as a half-dozen donuts. For example, the Caffé Vanilla Frappuccino has sixty-nine grams of sugar. The average donut at Dunkin' Donuts contains sixteen grams of sugar. In other words, that some coffees have the sugar equivalent of four and a half donuts at Dunkin' Donuts. It's an incredible amount of stimulant to be ingested in one sitting.

Keep in mind that the average cup of coffee has ninety-five to 200 grams of caffeine per eight-ounce cup.

Decaf Coffee

Contrary to what you may think, decaf coffee *does* contain caffeine. Decaf contains two to twelve milligrams per eight-ounce cup. By switching to decaf, you are drastically reducing caffeine intake. However, if you have coronary issues, be aware that there are small amounts of caffeine in decaf.

Herbal Coffee

Herbal coffees are made from many different things, for example, dandelion and sassafras root. Herbal coffees contain anywhere from forty to 120 milligrams of caffeine per eight-ounce cup.

Roasted Grain Beverages

Roasted grain beverages are not really coffee but rather a grain-based beverage that tastes very much like coffee but contains no caffeine whatsoever. They are made from grains such as barley and chicory and have molasses and other natural flavor enhancers added.

Yerba Mate

This drink has been popular in South America for centuries. It's an herbal tea made from the yerba plant. It tastes like coffee and is rich in antioxidants; it contains thirty to sixty milligrams of caffeine per eight-ounce cup.

Matcha

Matcha is a finely ground green tea leaf. It's a bright-green or emerald color. It's rich in antioxidants, polyphenols, chlorophyll, fiber, and vitamin C. According to experts, one cup of matcha has the nutritional equivalent of three to ten brewed green tea cups. Matcha contains between ten and thirty milligrams of caffeine per eight-ounce cup. Given its potent concentration of antioxidants, matcha is a good choice for anyone with kidney or liver disease, or elevated blood sugar, triglyceride, or cholesterol levels.

Green Tea

Chock full of antioxidants and packing ten to thirty milligrams of caffeine per eight-ounce cup, green tea is a real alternative to traditional coffee. Some of the benefits include evidence that green tea reduces the risk of heart disease, lowers blood pressure, reduces cholesterol levels, reduces inflammation, improves bone density, and helps neutralize free radicals that may be related to cancer.

Herbal Tea

Herbal teas are familiar to most people and come in all flavors—ginger, peppermint, orange, and many others. Most herbal teas contain about ten to thirty milligrams of caffeine per eight-ounce cup. So if you are looking to reduce or eliminate your caffeine intake, make sure to read the label of your favorite tea.

Black Tea

Black tea contains a substance called theophylline, which can speed up your heart rate and make you feel more alert. Black tea is also full of healthy substances called polyphenols, which are antioxidants that can help protect your cells from DNA damage. The average black tea has anywhere from forty to 120 milligrams per eight-ounce cup. If you are looking for less caffeine, be sure to read the label before consuming.

Chai Latte

Chai teas have their roots in the ancient Ayurvedic tradition of India. Chai teas are usually made from black tea mixed with traditional Indian herbs and spices, sweetened, and mixed with milk or a nondairy alternative. Chai latte varies in caffeine content, anywhere from forty to 120 milligrams per eight-ounce cup.

Your Love Affair with Chocolate

You do not have to give up chocolate as some recovery nutrition advocates suggest. Rather, you must be smarter about your chocolate intake. As long as you eat products that contain over 60 to 70 percent cocoa and partake of your favorite chocolate in moderation, you should have no issues. Many people ask why the percentage of cocoa matters. The higher the cocoa percentage, the higher the amount of real chocolate in the product. The lower the percentage of cocoa, the more it is a nonchocolate product and made with fillers such as high-fructose corn syrup. Strive to avoid any chocolate that is below the 70 percent cocoa threshold. If you don't like the taste of higher-cocoa-content chocolate, mix it with chocolate made from a lower-percentage chocolate until you adapt to the taste.

A 100-gram bar of dark chocolate with 70 percent cocoa or more contains eleven grams of fiber and the following percentages of the RDA for vitally important minerals: 67 percent for iron, 58 percent for magnesium, 89 percent for copper, and 98 percent for manganese. Chocolate also contains high levels of potassium, phosphorus, zinc, and selenium. Real chocolate can be good for you and a healthy snack.

Other Nutritional Recommendations and Tools
Thirty-Second Cracker Test

The saliva in your mouth can tell you a lot about how your body breaks down carbohydrates. Saliva contains enzymes, most notably amylase, which is responsible for breaking down food. Depending on your genetics, your saliva contains differing amounts of enzymes. Those with more amylase break down carbs faster, while those with less amylase break down carbs more slowly. It helps to have a rough idea of how your body breaks down carbs. You can integrate this information into your overall Spiritual Adrenaline nutritional plan.

To conduct this test, you need one saltine cracker (unsalted) or, for those who are sensitive to gluten, a gluten-free cracker or a dime-sized piece of raw potato and a watch or timer. When you are ready, put the cracker in your mouth and do not chew or swallow. Let the cracker sit in your mouth and let the enzymes in your saliva begin their work. Keep careful track of the time. You are waiting for the point where you sense a sweet taste. When you sense the sweetness, write down how long it took. Perform the cracker test two more times and average the time it took to taste the change and sense the sweetness. There are three major levels for how fast we digest carbs:

- Full: 0 to 14 seconds
- Moderate: 15 to 30 seconds
- Restricted: more than 30 seconds

If you are in the full category, you burn carbs fast and can have a larger percentage of your daily intake in carbs. If you are in the moderate category, you are in the midrange for carb burning and should be cautious about carb intake. If you are in the restricted category, you burn carbs slowly and need to really be aware of your carb intake, as your body does not have the ability to burn carbs off as efficiently as others.

There are many reasons why people in recovery should cut back on carbohydrate intake. This test is important, as it may confirm for you why your body had a harder time breaking down carbs from alcohol than others and why you add on pounds more easily than others.

Calorie-Counting Apps

There are so many free apps you can download to help you keep track of your calories or know what you are about to consume beforehand. I recommend Diet Assistant, Calorie King, and Weight Watchers Mobile. Some of these apps will let you use your smart phone to scan the UPC code on a product when you are out shopping. This helps you make healthier choices. If you eat clean, which means a diet composed almost exclusively of real food, you really don't need to worry about calories. You can eat all the green veggies you want, and the same is true for lean protein sources. Since these foods do not provide a dopamine rush the way sugar- and starch-based foods do, we tend to self-regulate with these foods and will stop eating when we are full. It's when we eat sugars, starches, processed foods, or ultrafatty sauces that we need to start watching calories.

For example, let's say you are at McDonald's and order a salad. The salad dressing likely contains a relatively large amount of fat. The Southwest Salad Dressing packet (44 milliliters) contains one gram of saturated fat and eight grams of total fat. That's a lot for such a small amount of salad dressing. If an otherwise low-calorie and healthy food such as salmon is being prepared in butter, it also becomes much higher in calories and fat. So it's important to know how foods are prepared and the nutritional content of salad dressing and other sauces.

Stress Eating

Anticipating a highly stressful day in advance permits you to prepare for the stress with filling and nutritious foods. These foods will help you cope with stress by providing your brain with the nutrients it needs to prompt the production of healthy hormones, while avoiding the production of cortisol and helping you function optimally. If you anticipate a stressful day, pack healthy complex carbs to avoid grabbing for junk, and stick to frequent smaller meals every two-and-a-half to three hours. The more you stay with healthy choices, the less appealing the junk or fast food will become. Trust me!

Plan B

Always have a protein or fruit-and-nut bar with you in case you are running late or have a change in plans. In order to have a healthy alternative, before you leave to go on the road, train, bus, or airplane, simply grab a bar or mix some protein powder with water, take it with you, and enjoy it, and your hunger will go away. This way, you avoid the alternative of grabbing fast food, such as a burger, chips, fries, or fried chicken, undercutting all your hard work.

Spiritual Adrenaline Inspiration: Alex F., Massachusetts

Alex F. is a kiteboarding and surfing instructor based in Cape Cod, Massachusetts. He has six-plus years in recovery. His drugs of choice were alcohol and marijuana.

When Alex was eleven years old, he was diagnosed with dyslexia. As a child and even now as an adult, Alex has difficulty communicating through writing. Reflecting on his childhood, he says that he "made a decision to never trust my brain again." Rather than trust in himself and build self-confidence, he turned to the external world. As he did so, alcohol and weed became his primary coping mechanisms. As the years passed, Alex found that active addiction to alcohol and other drugs led him to give away the things he valued most in life: his friends, his family, his sanity, and his health.

> Much like the trust I have in my higher power, a commitment to nutrition and exercise has never let me down. The positive impact is guaranteed as long as I strive for growth and avoid the false promise of perfection. Being tuned into my nutrition and health prevents dramatic emotional slides. Being healthy helps me "take it easy." I find that anxiety, stress, and craving levels are inversely proportional to my level of bodily and spiritual heath. When I'm on the beam—holding close to my higher power's will for my life—I simply don't get acute or chronic attacks of stress, anxiety, and cravings that overwhelm me. That doesn't mean I don't get acute comfort food and sugar cravings, because I do. However, with application of the principles learned in the Twelve Steps, specifically a whole lot of prayer and meditation, these cravings don't dominate me for days.

Alex absolutely loves his life today. He teaches kiteboarding and surfing and has traveled the globe. Recently he traveled to Mexico to meet sober friends for some surfing action. He says that recovery has given him back all that he gave away to alcohol and drugs. He does all these things because "my higher power is crazy about me and loves to see me joyous. I no longer mistrust my brain but rather I endeavor to keep it quiet, strong, and focused."

Here is his advice to those interested in taking their recovery to the next level:

- Go one day with no refined sugar. Then go for two, and so on.
- Lose five pounds eating healthier, and then keep that weight off for a month. Then focus on the next five pounds.
- Exercise (walk, climb stairs) for ten minutes twice a day for a month. Then increase to fifteen minutes.
- Set easily achievable short-term goals.
- Be gentle with yourself.
- Remind yourself constantly that the images of perfect bodies and beauty we are bombarded with are not what we are after. We want to feel better and have more energy in our day-to-day life.
- No beating up on yourself if you fall short of your goals.
- Plan your meals and pack healthy snacks to avoid getting overly hungry and needing food quickly.
- Complex carbs and healthy fats are the key elements in long-term weight management. Protein is not an energy source for the body; it helps in muscular recovery and maintenance. Most people eat too much of it.
- Read labels. For example, instant oatmeal has large amounts of sodium; steel-cut, slow-cook oatmeal has none.
- Turn over control of your outside issues to your higher power.

CHAPTER NINE

Addiction Paleo and Recovery Superfoods

Almost everybody in active addiction is nutrient deficient.[152] This is true as well for those who are in active addiction and are obese, since the majority of calories come from foods with little nutritional value, most notably alcohol. However, comfort foods such as candy and soda can also contribute to malnourishment. For many in recovery, although they no longer use their drug of choice, their recovery lifestyle often continues with poor eating habits, lots of comfort foods, smoking, and dehydration caused by nicotine and excessive caffeine intake. So whether you're a newcomer or someone who has been in recovery for a while but has failed to focus on healthy diet and exercise, you are basically in the same nutrient-deficient state. Many in long-term recovery, with ten or more years, are similarly nutrient deficient.

Ketogenics vs. Paleo

A ketogenic diet is one with a maximum of 10 percent of your total daily calories from carbohydrates. People who are on a ketogenic diet get their energy primarily from healthy fat sources, for example, avocado and oily fish such as salmon. For people in recovery just beginning to modify their diet and focus on the self-care program in this book, I do not recommend going ketogenic.

Your body needs antioxidants and other nutrients to heal after years of substance abuse. If you are a smoker, you continue to put stress on internal organs, as each cigarette fills your lungs and bloodstream with toxins.

On my Addiction Paleo plan (I'll share about that later), approximately 30 percent of your calories come from healthy carb sources, almost all complex carbs. This includes a wide range of antioxidants, flavonoids, and other nutrients that will restore your body to health.

I am a fan of short-term ketogenic diets, for example, to detox off sugar. However, I believe ketogenic diets are dangerous if continued in the long term. My opinion rests on the fact that while people on a ketogenic diet may feel an abundance of energy from taking in healthy fats, they exclude other nutrients, antioxidants being the perfect example, that the body needs to neutralize cancer-causing free radicals and other toxins.

Having been on numerous ketogenic diets over the years for training purposes, I can tell you from experience that my body was not able to deal with the stress of my personal and professional life for more than a week to ten days. At times, I felt the diet actually *caused* my body stress when I stayed ketogenic for more than a week to ten days. I realize ketogenic diets are popular right now, and you may be skeptical about the "dangers" of a ketogenic diet. Many people are going ketogenic, and a number of prominent authors have written best-selling books espousing the virtues of this type of diet. There are myriad research papers and discussions about this subject on the internet, which is not always the ideal resource to get information. However, before going ketogenic you should read the scientific research and other information available and make your own informed decision. I encourage you to consult with your doctor or other trusted medical professional before you try a ketogenic or paleo diet.

Addiction Paleo

My Addiction Paleo plan takes into account how your substance abuse damaged your nutrient retention, hormone creation, and organ health. I don't go into what percentage of your calories should come from carbohydrates; that's complicated and hard to remember. Instead, Addiction Paleo recommends an early-afternoon "carb cutoff." In my program, you can eat complex carbs in moderation from the time you wake up until lunchtime. After lunch, carb intake is heavily restricted. As people with a history of substance abuse, our diet needs antioxidants and complex carbohydrates in larger amounts than that of the general population.

Rather than set ratios or percentages of carbohydrates, proteins, and fats you should take in, Addiction Paleo focuses on the time of the day. In the early part of the day, I suggest you eat more carbs and proteins, and include some fat. As the day progresses, shift to consuming more proteins and fat and fewer carbs. In the late afternoon or early evening, eliminate carbs and focus on proteins and fats.

Addiction Paleo takes into account your history of substance abuse and research on how these substances impact nutrient retention and hormone creation in the body. I suggest you add antioxidants and complex carbohydrates to slowly restore your body to health. Spiritual Adrenaline focuses on cancer-fighting antioxidants that neutralize free radicals, reduce inflammation, and stabilize blood sugar to lessen depression, mood swings, and cravings.[153] I even offer suggestions, subject to your doctor's approval, on specific foods for those of you with common health concerns created by substance abuse, including foods for people with liver disease, early-stage heart disease, kidney and/or pancreas disease, and smoking-related lung disease.

Diet alone cannot cure these conditions, but there are specific foods that can help your body heal, as well as some to avoid. One easy example is the elimination of high-fructose corn syrup, especially for those with compromised liver function or liver disease.[154] Liver disease makes it more difficult to break down high-fructose corn syrup, which is a cheap filler in many foods and almost all processed sweet comfort foods and candy. The syrup accumulates in your liver and causes added stress and inflammation.[155]

Reduction of Inflammation

Inflammation is your body's way of protecting itself from infection, illness, or injury. As part of this process, your white blood cell count increases along with other substances to help fight the perceived infection or illness. Long-term exposure to anxiety and stress can cause inflammation. Just because you cannot see it on the outside does not mean it's not happening on the inside. Diseases that are associated with chronic inflammation include fatty liver, diabetes, and heart disease. Addiction Paleo seeks to reduce inflammation through dietary modification. Foods that cause inflammation include those with high amounts of sugar and high-fructose corn syrup, processed carbs such as white bread, foods with trans fats such as processed pastries and candies and other sweets, and alcohol.[156] Lack of physical exercise is also a major cause of inflammation.

The foods that are integrated into my Addiction Paleo plan include nature's inflammation-reducing superfoods and spices. First, you will incorporate much-needed antioxidants to fight off inflammation and cancer-causing free radicals. Second, you will learn to balance macronutrients, carbs, proteins, and healthy fats to levels consistent with those that research has confirmed reduce inflammation. Third, you will incorporate fun and doable exercise and "active fellowship" to activate your body's internal fat-burning, hormone-producing, and inflammation-fighting mechanisms. Active fellowship includes such things as walking around the block with others in recovery or more intense activities such as hiking, weight training, CrossFit, and yoga.

Medium-Chain Triglycerides (Fatty Acids)

Medium-chain triglycerides, or MCTs, have many health benefits. They are found naturally in coconut and palm oil. The chemical structure of MCTs makes them easier than other fats to metabolize in the liver.[157] The ease and speed with which MCTs can be broken down benefits anyone with compromised liver function or liver disease. The speed at which MCTs break down provides two additional benefits. First, MCTs provide a more immediate source of energy since they metabolize and enter the bloodstream faster than other types of healthy fats.[158] Second, studies have also confirmed that MCTs make weight loss easier, as they can easily and quickly be broken down by the body. This makes it less likely that MCTs go unused and be converted into fat cells that add weight and harm your health.

MCTs are also great to take the "edge off" when you are cutting back on carbs. Your brain can get energy from two sources: glucose and MCTs. So as you reduce your carb intake, the amount of glucose available for brain function drops and you may start to crave carbs. Work in a teaspoon of MCTs, and your brain has what it needs to function. This helps take the edge off relatively quickly and makes cutting carbs easier.

Reduction of Pharmaceuticals and Increase in Nutritional Therapy

As the opiate epidemic has driven home, the use of opiates, benzos, and other pharmaceutical "solutions" to medical issues often comes with horrific consequences. For some, the cure is worse than the disease and can turn a nondeadly disease into a prescription addiction that for some will lead to death. Pharmaceuticals can also cause stress to internal organs already weakened and damaged by long-term substance abuse. Ketogenic and paleo diets have been used since the 1920s to treat certain conditions and may sometimes eliminate the need for prescribed medication.[159] This is most true for those with hypoglycemia or type 2 diabetes. This is also true for those with respiratory and cardiovascular disease, which also disproportionately impacts members of the recovery community.[160]

Integration of Exercise and Breath

Exercise is an important piece of the Addiction Paleo program, as are the nutrients you eat that prime your body to perform at optimal efficiency. Exercise assists the body in the natural process of breaking down and absorbing nutrients more efficiently, eliminating waste and toxic substances, dramatically reducing inflammation, and prompting the creation of important hormones. Deep inhaling and exhaling, whether while meditating or during exercise, also aids the process of healing in the body. Deep breaths ensure that fresh, oxygen-rich blood gets to cells throughout your body and permits your organs to better perform metabolic functions.

The following list includes my top recovery superfoods. These foods contain a large amount of other vitamins and minerals in addition to those presented here. I'm focusing on the benefits of foods that contain specific nutrients, helping to restore the vitamins and minerals you as a person in recovery need. *It's helpful to think of food not just as something pleasurable, something to stuff yourself with in order to fill emotional voids in your life, but rather as a recovery tool that can help you achieve long-term health and happiness in recovery.*

It's good to keep these foods in mind as you begin your journey. Get to know them, as they are nature's medicine and will help restore you to health.

Recovery Superfoods

Food	Contains	Benefits
Vegetables		
Asparagus	Folate; potassium; selenium; thiamine; calcium; vitamins A, B, C, E, K; copper; phosphorus	Energy, mood, hormone production, blood-sugar stabilization, antioxidants; promotes heart health, acts as a diuretic, and aids in detox and cleansing process
Avocado	Glutamine; vitamins B6, C, E, K; folic acid; mood; pantothenic acid; glutathione; copper; magnesium; potassium; lutein; beta-carotene; omega-3	Energy, hormone production, mood, blood-sugar stabilization; promotes absorption of antioxidants
Beets	Fiber, protein, folate, manganese, potassium, copper, magnesium, iron, vitamins C and B	Antioxidants, energy, blood-sugar stabilization, healthy nerve and muscle function; promotes health of bones, liver, kidneys, and pancreas
Broccoli	Vitamins A, B1, C, E, K; folate; chromium; riboflavin; potassium; fiber; copper; protein; zinc; iron; selenium; choline; indole;, thiocyanotes	Energy, mood, hormone production, blood-sugar stabilization, antioxidants; promotes detox of liver, kidneys, and pancreas
Brussels Sprouts	Vitamins A, B6, C, K; folate; potassium; manganese; fiber; choline; copper; phosphorus; omega-3 fatty acids; glucoraphanin; glucobrassin; sinigrin; gluconasturtiin; iron	Energy, mood, hormone production blood-sugar stabilization, fiber, antioxidants
Carrots	Fiber; vitamins A, B6, K1; potassium; beta-carotene; alpha-carotene; lutein; lycopene; polyacetylenese; anthocyanins	Energy, mood, hormone production, blood-sugar stabilization, antioxidants; detox of liver, kidneys; heart healthy, lowers bad cholesterol, eye health
Cauliflower	Vitamins, C, K, B6, B12; folate; fiber; thiamine; riboflavin; niacin; magnesium; protein; thiamine; phosphorus; pantothenic acid; potassium; manganese; glucosinolates	Energy, mood, hormone production, blood-sugar stabilization, anti-inflammatory; supports detox of liver, kidneys, and pancreas
Collard Greens	Vitamins A, C, K; choline; calcium; magnesium	Energy, mood, hormone production, blood-sugar stabilization

Food	Contains	Benefits
Garlic	Allicin; pantothenic acid; riboflavin; thiamine; Vitamins A, B6, C, E, K; potassium; calcium; copper; iron; magnesium; manganese; selenium; zinc; phosphorus	Energy, mood, hormone production, blood-sugar stabilization; lowers blood pressure; antioxidant; supports detox of liver, kidneys, pancreas
Green Peas	Manganese, fiber, thiamine, copper, vitamins B6 and C; niacin, riboflavin, zinc, magnesium, iron, potassium, choline, phosphorus, folate	Energy, mood, hormone production, blood-sugar stabilization
Kale	Vitamins A, C, E, K; copper; potassium; calcium; phosphorus; iron	Energy, mood, hormone production, blood-sugar stabilization, fiber; high in vitamin K, antioxidants; anti-inflammatory; supports heart health; good source of calcium
Mushrooms	Copper, selenium, riboflavin, potassium, zinc, thiamine, manganese, choline, folate, phosphorus, calcium	Energy, mood, hormone production, blood-sugar stabilization; helps lower blood pressure, supports immune system
Parsley	Vitamins A, C, K; folate; iron; zeaxanthin; potassium; magnesium; beta-carotene	Energy, mood, antioxidants, bone health, heart health, blood-sugar stabilization
Spinach	Potassium, vitamins A and E, manganese, folate, iron, free-form amino acids, l-glutamine, folic acid	Energy, mood, hormone production, blood-sugar stabilization, muscle growth
Sweet Potato	Beta-carotene; vitamins A, B6, C, E; potassium; manganese; calcium; iron; magnesium; phosphorus; zinc; thiamine; riboflavin; folate; carotenoids	Energy, mood, hormone production, blood-sugar stabilization, brain and organ function, hormone production
Tomatoes	Vitamins A, C, K; folic acid; copper; potassium; beta-carotene; lutein; biotin	Energy, mood, hormone production, blood-sugar stabilization, antioxidants
Watercress	Lutein; zeaxanthin; protein; folate; pantothenic acid; copper; vitamins A, B6, C, E, K; thiamine; riboflavin; calcium; magnesium; phosphorus; potassium	Energy, mood, hormone production, blood-sugar stabilization, lung function; detox of liver, kidneys, and pancreas; lowers blood pressure

Food	Contains	Benefits
Fruit		
Apples	Khellin, vitamins A and C, dietary fiber, flavonoids, polyphenols, pantothenic acid, phosphorus, iron, calcium, pectin	Antioxidants, energy, blood-sugar stabilization; reduces risk of cancer, heart disease, hypertension, and diabetes
Blueberries	Resveratrol, gallic acid, lutein, zeaxanthin, vitamins K and C, manganese, fiber, potassium, folate, antioxidants, phytonutrients, phenols, anthocyanins	Antioxidants, energy, blood-sugar stabilization; lowers cholesterol; promotes heart and skin health
Cantaloupe	Thiamine, vitamins A and K, niacin, magnesium, ester-C	Antioxidants, energy; promotes insulin and blood sugar metabolism; reduces oxidative stress in kidneys and improves insulin resistance
Cranberries	Fiber; manganese; vitamins C, E, K; copper; pantothenic acid; beta-carotene; lutein; zeaxanthin	Anti-inflammatory, antioxidants; supports immune system; promotes heart health; detoxes liver, kidneys, and pancreas; energy; fiber
Goji Berries	Antioxidants, zinc, iron, fiber, vitamins A and C	Antioxidants, energy, blood-sugar stabilization; improves immune system function; detoxifies the liver
Grapefruit	Fiber; vitamins A, B1, B5, C; potassium; biotin; antioxidants	Antioxidants, energy, blood-sugar stabilization; promotes cardiovascular health by lowering triglycerides; skin and lung health
Kiwi	Linoleic acid; choline; potassium; iron; vitamins A, B6, C; fiber	Antioxidants (more vitamin C than other fruits), blood-sugar stabilization; helps with sleep; promotes digestion and healthy skin
Lemon	Fiber (pectin), vitamin B6 and C, potassium, citric acid	Fiber, antioxidants, kidney health, cardiovascular health, blood-sugar stabilization; helps reduce inflammation

Food	Contains	Benefits
Papaya	Vitamins A and C, folate, fiber, magnesium, potassium, copper, pantothenic acid, lutein, zeaxanthin, lycopene, beta-carotene, papain, polyphenols	Antioxidants, blood-sugar stabilization; detoxifies liver, kidneys, and pancreas; reduces inflammation; energy; promotes digestion and breakdown of proteins; stress reduction
Pomegranate	Vitamins C and K, folate, potassium, protein, fiber, punicalagins, punicic acid	Antioxidants, blood-sugar stabilization; detoxes liver, kidneys and pancreas; reduces inflammation; promotes energy; lowers blood pressure
Pumpkin	Fiber; potassium; vitamins A, C, B6, E; riboflavin; potassium; copper; manganese; thiamine; folate; pantothenic acid; niacin; iron; magnesium; phosphorus	Antioxidants; supports heart health; detoxifies liver, kidneys and pancreas; supports immune system; energy; good source of fiber
Raspberries	Vitamins C, E, K; biotin; potassium; magnesium; copper; ellagic acid	Antioxidants, energy, blood-sugar stabilization; promotes heart, liver, and skin health
Strawberries	Vitamin C, potassium, fiber, iodine, folate, copper, potassium, magnesium	Antioxidants, energy, blood-sugar stabilization; promotes heart, liver, and kidney health; fights depression, hypertension, allergies, and asthma
Watermelon	Vitamins A, B6, C; lycopene; potassium; antioxidants; amino acids	Antioxidants, energy, blood-sugar stabilization; fights asthma; promotes health of cardiovascular system, digestive system; muscle recovery; skin health

Seeds, Nuts, and Beans

Food	Contains	Benefits
Almonds	Vitamin E, biotin, manganese, phosphorus, fiber, monounsaturated fats, phenols, flavonoids, phenolic acid, polyphenols, tyrosine, protein	Antioxidants, blood- sugar stabilization; promotes cardiovascular health and lower cholesterol levels; assists with weight loss; energy
Black Beans	Protein, iron, copper, manganese, thiamine, phosphorus, magnesium, folic acid	Healthy bones; promotes cardiovascular health; lowers blood pressure; assists in stabilizing blood-sugar levels; promotes weight loss; energy

Food	Contains	Benefits
Cashews	Copper, phosphorus, manganese, zinc, magnesium, lutein, zeaxanthin, oleic acid, protein	Heart health; excellent source of copper, fiber; stabilizes blood sugar; energy
Chia Seeds	Omega-3 fatty acids, fiber, protein, iron, calcium, magnesium, zinc	Helps raise good cholesterol; blood–sugar stabilization, heart health, fiber
Chickpeas	Fiber, protein, manganese, folate, copper, phosphorus, iron, zinc, selenium, calcium, protein	Stabilizes blood sugar; lowers blood pressure; promotes cardiovascular health, bone health; reduces inflammation; promotes weight loss
Flaxseed	Omega-3, magnesium, tryptophan, thiamine, linoleic acid, vitamins B1 and E, fiber, protein, selenium, phosphorus	High in fiber, low in carbs; detoxifies the colon; promotes fat loss; reduces cravings for sugar; promotes skin and hair health; lowers cholesterol; antioxidants, energy
Fennel	Flavonoid antioxidants, fiber, niacin, pyridoxine, riboflavin, thiamin, vitamins A and C, potassium, calcium, copper, iron, magnesium, phosphorus, zinc	Antioxidants, fiber; assists in detox of kidneys, liver, and pancreas; assists in lowering blood pressure; promotes stable blood sugar; boosts immune system
Garbanzo Beans	Protein, fiber, manganese, folate, copper, phosphorus, iron, zinc, calcium, potassium, zinc, selenium, vitamins K and B6, thiamine, riboflavin, pantothenic acid, flavonoids	Antioxidants; promotes cardiovascular health; stabilizes blood sugar; promotes skin health and weight loss; boosts immune system; good protein source
Lentils	Iron, folate, fiber, copper, phosphorus, thiamine, zinc, vitamin B6, manganese, potassium, protein	Promotes cardiovascular and digestive health; stabilizes blood sugar; good protein source; boosts energy levels; promotes weight loss
Pecans	More than nineteen vitamins and minerals	Anti-inflammatory; stabilizes blood sugar; reduces hypertension; promotes weight loss; promotes cardiovascular and skin health; strengthens immune system

Food	Contains	Benefits
Pistachios	Monounsaturated fatty acids, lutein, beta-carotene, vitamin E	Antioxidants; stabilizes blood sugar; high in fiber; improves digestive health; promotes cardiovascular and skin health
Peanuts	Vitamins B6 and E, magnesium, potassium, monounsaturated fats	Reduces risk of heart disease, diabetes; stabilizes blood sugar; boosts immune system; promotes weight loss; high protein content
Pumpkin Seeds	Beta-carotene, beta-cryptoxanthin, tyrosine, tryptophan, lutein, linoleic acid, vitamin E, magnesium, copper, protein, zinc, phytosterols, omega-3	Promotes cardiovascular health, boosts immune system, contains healthy fat, stabilizes blood sugar, promotes liver health and sleep; anti-inflammatory
Sunflower Seeds	Vitamins B1, B6, E; folate; copper; manganese; selenium; phosphorus; magnesium	Promotes cardiovascular health, reduces inflammation, stabilizes blood sugar, reduces hypertension; high in antioxidants; supports bone, skin, and muscle health
Wheat Germ	Vitamin B6, linoleic acid, choline	Promotes cardiovascular health; anti-inflammatory; boosts immune system; supports bone, skin, and muscle health; stabilizes blood sugar
Walnuts	Omega-3 fats, copper, manganese, molybdenum, biotin, L-arginine, numerous antioxidants	Promotes cardiovascular health; anti-inflammatory; reduces hypertension; promotes weight loss; stabilizes blood sugar

Protein Sources

Food	Contains	Benefits
Fish	Tryptophan and 5-HTP, thiamine, tyrosine, folic acid, niacin, branched-chain amino acids, choline, pantothenic acid, creatine, vitamin D, protein, BCAA	Omega-3 fatty acids; promotes cardiovascular health; promotes brain health and function; improves mood; natural source of vitamin D; may help prevent asthma and type 1 diabetes; improves sleep; stabilizes blood sugar

Food	Contains	Benefits
Lean Meats (grass fed)	Beta-carotene, vitamins B and E, thiamin, riboflavin, calcium, magnesium, potassium, omega-3, protein, BCAA	Lean protein; promotes healthy red blood cell production; boosts energy; promotes cardiovascular health; can contribute to stabilizing blood sugar
Turkey	Protein, iron, zinc, potassium, phosphorus, vitamin B6, niacin, tryptophan and other amino acids, selenium, BCAA	Lean protein; promotes cardiovascular health; stabilizes blood sugar; contributes to stable insulin levels; helps sleep; boosts immune system
Soybeans	Protein, copper, manganese, phosphorus, iron, riboflavin, magnesium, vitamins B and K, potassium, calcium, copper, iron	Lean protein, appetite suppression; boosts metabolic function; improves digestive and bone health; helps to lower cholesterol levels; aids in maintaining weight and stabilizing blood sugar; promotes cardiovascular, bone, and digestive health; promotes healthy sleep
Eggs	Choline; selenium; protein; vitamins B2, B5, B12, D; phosphorus; riboflavin; many essential amino acids including leucine; zinc; calcium; BCAA	Lean protein, cardiovascular health; aids in liver function; brain health; muscle growth and retention
Carbs		
Brown Rice	Vitamins B1, B3, B6; magnesium; thiamine; niacin; iron; phosphorus; dietary fiber; selenium; copper	Sustains energy, brain and organ function, mood; assists with muscle growth and maintenance; blood-sugar stabilization; hormone production; low glycemic load
Quinoa	Protein (complete including lysine), amino acids, fiber, iron, magnesium, riboflavin (B2), manganese, flavonoids, quercetin, kaempferol	High in protein, gluten free, all essential amino acids, low glycemic load; boosts metabolic health; high in antioxidants; can promote weight loss
Whole-Grain Bread	Fiber, iron, magnesium, selenium, protein, vitamin B, antioxidants, zinc, copper, magnesium	Cardiovascular health, low glycemic load; stabilizes blood sugar; can promote weight loss

Food	Contains	Benefits
Ezekiel Bread	Protein, fiber, vitamin B1, phosphorus, magnesium, niacin, all nine essential amino acids	Cardiovascular health, low glycemic load; helps stabilize blood sugar; gluten free
Tapioca Bread	Fiber, low in sugar, low in calories	Cardiovascular health, low glycemic load, gluten free; helps stabilize blood sugar
Coconut Bread	Fiber, low in sugar, healthy fats, low in calories	Cardiovascular health, low glycemic load, gluten free; helps stabilize blood sugar
Oils		
Coconut Oil	MCFA (caprylic, lauric, capric acids), antioxidants	Promotes heart health, lowers bad and increases good cholesterol, promotes liver health, reduces inflammation, provides energy, promotes health of pancreas
Extra Virgin Olive Oil	Antioxidants, healthy fats, fewer free radicals, oleic acid, polyphenols	Antioxidants; promotes heart health; reduces inflammation; helps lower blood pressure and stabilize blood sugar
Beverages		
Apple Cider	Pectin; vitamins B1, B2, B6, C; biotin; folic acid	Boosts energy, stabilizes blood sugar; detox of liver, kidneys; heart healthy; mood enhancer
Vinegar	Niacin, pantothenic acid, sodium, phosphorus, potassium, calcium, iron, magnesium	See apple cider
Green Tea	Vitamins A, B, C, E; polyphenols and other antioxidants; catechins; chlorophyll; amino acids; theanine (amino acid)	Antioxidants; stabilizes blood sugar; helps lower cholesterol; promotes heart, liver, and kidney health
Dandelion Tea	Vitamins A, B6, C, K; calcium; iron; magnesium; potassium; fiber; antioxidants	Supports bone and heart health; one dandelion contains over 500% of the daily allowance for vitamin K; cleanses the liver; stabilizes blood sugar; high in antioxidants; reduces inflammation

Food	Contains	Benefits
Matcha	Vitamins A, B, C, E; polyphenols and other antioxidants; catechins; chlorophyll; amino acids; theanine (amino acid)	Same as green tea except multiplied by 3 to 10 times
Light Roast Coffee	Antioxidants, chlorogenic acid	Heart, liver, kidney health; anti oxidants; reduces inflammation; stabilizes blood sugar
Water	None, but necessary to break down and carry nutrients to cells and for almost all other functions at the cellular level	Necessary for all body functions
Condiments		
Sea Salt	Electrolytes, over 60 trace minerals	Supports brain, lung, heart, muscle, and nervous system function
Black Pepper	Manganese, vitamin K, copper, fiber, calcium, chromium, iron	Anti-inflammatory; helps stabilize blood sugar; lung health; antioxidant
Vegetable Ketchup	Depends on brand and specific veggies used	No high-fructose corn syrup, and benefits of vegetables used
Dijon Mustard	Folate, vitamin A, potassium, calcium, phosphorus, magnesium, fiber	Lung health; lowers cholesterol; stabilizes blood sugar; heart health; antioxidants; promotes detox of organs; no high-fructose corn syrup
Spicy Mustard	Very similar to Dijon but varies depending on spices	See Dijon. Depends on spices used. No high-fructose corn syrup
Hot Sauce	Varies depending on spices used	No high-fructose corn syrup, and benefits of spices used
Various:		
Dark Chocolate (cocoa 70% or more)	Manganese, copper, antioxidants, flavanol, iron, phosphorus, potassium, zinc, selenium, calcium, vitamin K	Lowers blood pressure, lowers good cholesterol, promotes heart health, reduces inflammation; promotes heart, kidney, and liver health; stabilizes blood sugar

For People with Liver Disease

If you have liver damage from long-term alcohol abuse, hepatitis, or any other issues, you need to consult with your doctor before adopting any of the recommended nutritional advice in this book. People with liver damage have a difficult time processing protein. When protein cannot be processed, it builds up in the liver and can become toxic.[161] In consultation with your doctor, you may want to come up with a plan to reduce protein or substitute plant-based proteins for animal-based proteins, since plant-based proteins are easier to digest.[162] You may also want to increase complex carbohydrates beyond what is otherwise recommended in this book to assist your liver to function and to facilitate the breakdown of proteins and other nutrients.

Fatty Liver

Poor nutrition and abuse of alcohol and other substances contribute to fatty liver.[163] The result is that fat tissue starts to build up in the liver. When the fat in your liver makes up 5 percent or more of liver tissue, the condition is known as fatty liver. This can cause inflammation and scarring of the liver. Over 90 percent of the fifteen million people in the United States who abuse alcohol eventually develop fatty liver.[164] Fatty liver can even occur after a short period of heavy drinking in what is known as acute alcoholic liver disease.

Liver disease related to alcohol consumption fits into one of three categories: fatty liver, alcoholic hepatitis, or cirrhosis.[165] Cocaine use and the use of other drugs can also cause organ damage, which impacts proper functions of the organs.[166] Fatty liver is generally reversible with abstinence, and it is not believed to predispose a person to chronic liver disease if abstinence is maintained.[167] Alcoholic hepatitis is a form of alcohol-induced liver injury that occurs with the consumption of large quantities of alcohol over a prolonged period of time. Cirrhosis involves replacement of the normal tissues with scars or thick bands of fibrous tissue, which can result in liver failure.[168] Only you and your doctor can determine the extent of the damage to your liver—and the lifestyle changes that are appropriate for you. This remarkable organ has the ability to regenerate healthy tissue in many cases. Simple changes to diet and lifestyle can greatly aid in the healing process.

Foods That Cleanse the Liver

If you are looking to detox your liver, with your doctor's approval, here are some foods that will help you.

Garlic

Garlic's medicinal qualities are derived from its high amount of allicin and selenium. These compounds are widely recognized as helpful in cleansing the liver as it forces out toxins.

Beets and Carrots

High in plant flavonoids including catechins and beta-carotene, these vegetables stimulate overall liver function. Flavonoids are a nutrient group found in plants, fruits, and vegetables that have powerful antioxidant qualities. Catechins are among the most recommended flavonoids.

Green Tea

Also full of catechins, green tea is widely recognized to contribute to liver health, lower cholesterol, and possibly reduce the risk of heart disease and cancer.

Avocado

Avocado prompts the body to produce glutathione, a compound necessary for your liver to cleanse itself of harmful toxins.

Apples

Pectin in apples enhances your body's ability to produce enzymes necessary to cleanse the liver and excrete toxins from the digestive tract. Apples are also high in anti-inflammatory compounds and fiber.

Leafy Green Vegetables

High in plant chlorophyllase, leafy greens absorb toxins from the bloodstream and also can neutralize toxins.

Broccoli and Cauliflower

These two vegetables contain indoles, thiocyanates, and glucosinolate; these substances enhance enzyme production in the liver and help flush out carcinogens and toxins. Both are high in vitamin C.

Cabbage

Cabbage is packed full of phytochemicals that break up free radicals. It is also high in vitamins B, C, and K and folic acid (B vitamin).

Olive Oil

A great source of oleic acid and monounsaturated fat, olive oil is also rich in polyphenols and antioxidants, which neutralize free radicals. Virgin or extra virgin olive oil is generally higher in antioxidants.

Coconut Oil

Full of medium-chain amino acids, coconut oil metabolizes quickly in the liver. It also lessens stress on your liver and reduces inflammation.

TUDCA

This is not a food but rather a bile acid that can be taken as a supplement that provides relief to a damaged or overstressed liver. Tauroursodeoxycholic acid, commonly referred to as TUDCA, is a bile acid, produced in and released by the gallbladder, that helps digest fat. Researchers have confirmed many other roles that TUDCA can play in improving your health. For example, TUDCA can increase insulin sensitivity, combat liver cirrhosis, and treat hepatitis and certain complications of diabetes.[169]

For People with Heart Disease

Some people are born with heart health–related issues that are handed down through genes. But for most, lifestyle rather than genetics contributes to heart disease.

My initial blood test with Dr. Michael Bedecs confirmed that I had a five times increased risk of heart disease based upon the markers (triglycerides) in my blood. That got my attention. The US Centers for Disease Control lists the following lifestyle factors as the leading causes of heart disease:

unhealthy diet, physical inactivity, obesity, too much alcohol, and smoking. The good news is that the lifestyle changes recommended in the Spiritual Adrenaline program empower you to change your lifestyle to lower your risk. Here are some heart-healthy foods[170] I recommend. As with starting any lifestyle change, you should get your doctor's sign-off before beginning.

Foods That Are Heart Healthy

Salmon

Salmon and other "oily" fish like sardines and mackerel should be a part of a heart-healthy diet. These fish are high in omega-3 and 6.

Oatmeal

Oatmeal is high in soluble fiber that can lower cholesterol. The soluble fiber acts like a sponge in the digestive tract and absorbs cholesterol so it can be eliminated from, rather than absorbed into, the bloodstream.

Berries

Blueberries, cranberries, raspberries, and other berries contain anthocyanins and flavonoids.

Dark Chocolate

Dark chocolate contains flavonoids known as polyphenols, which have been shown to help reduce blood pressure, clotting, and inflammation. Dark chocolate means more than 70 percent is cocoa.

Tomatoes

Tomatoes contain the antioxidant lycopene. Lycopene is a carotenoid that can help lower the amount of "bad cholesterol" to help keep blood vessels open and avoid clotting.

Nuts

Almonds, walnuts, pistachios, and macadamia nuts all contain the highest amount of cholesterol-lowering fiber. They also contain vitamin E, which helps lower cholesterol. Walnuts are a particularly good choice as they are high in omega-3 fatty acids.

Avocado

Avocados are full of monounsaturated fat, the good kind, which has been shown to lower heart disease risk factors like high cholesterol levels. Avocados also contain antioxidants and potassium, both of which are important for heart health.

Extra Virgin Olive Oil

Extra virgin olive oil is an excellent source of monounsaturated fat.

Green Tea

Green tea is full of heart-healthy antioxidants.

For People with Kidney Disease

Your BUN[171] and creatinine levels are indicators of your overall kidney function and health. If your blood tests indicate kidney disease or damage, here are some nutritional recommendations.

I have intentionally selected foods that overlap to aid both liver and kidney cleansing. This will make incorporating healthy food choices into your diet much easier.

Foods That Cleanse the Kidneys

- Cabbage
- Garlic
- Broccoli, cauliflower
- Apples
- Olive oil
- Blueberries, cranberries, raspberries, strawberries

All are rich in phytonutrients, phenols, and anthocyanins, powerful antioxidants that assist in neutralizing toxins in the body.

The Pancreas

The pancreas has two main functions. First, it supplies enzymes that help to digest proteins, carbohydrates, and fats in your small intestine. Second, it secretes hormones, most notably insulin, that regulate your body's metabolism of sugar.[172] Abuse of alcohol and other drugs compromises the ability of the pancreas to function properly. If you have a compromised pancreas, the use of stimulants such as coffee or cigarettes must also be reduced or avoided. Insulin production can be harmed by poor nutrition choices such as eating foods full of unhealthy fats, especially trans fats, as well as high-carbohydrate diets.[173]

For Those with Pancreatic Disease

The National Pancreas Foundation recommends a low-fat diet. This means plant-based proteins as well as white fish like cod, bass, swordfish, and tilapia. For most people, it is recommended to restrict fat intake to below twenty grams of fat a day. Alcohol cannot be consumed safely, as it causes dehydration and makes the pancreas "flare."[174] Flares can be painful and promote inflammation because of the added stress to the pancreas and other organs.

Foods That Cleanse the Pancreas[175]

Yogurt

Live bacteria, also known as probiotics, in many yogurts help keep your digestive system balanced. Another alternative is kefir, which has a substantial number of probiotics.

Berries

Antioxidants in blueberries, strawberries, blackberries, and raspberries help neutralize free radicals.

Leafy Greens

Kale, spinach, and rhubarb are all high in the B vitamins that help the pancreas to function.

For People Who Smoke or Smoked

If you suffer from asthma, if you smoke, or if you have compromised lung function for any reason, modify your diet to mitigate the damage already done and to prevent future damage, including the greatest fear of every smoker—lung cancer. No single food or foods are a cure for any health concern, but my recommended list of foods can help your overall health by using nature's medicines, making the path to lifestyle change much easier. You cannot turn back the hands of time and make better decisions, but you can use the science available to you to promote the highest degree of lung health possible, despite your smoking history.

Smokers must focus on increasing the intake of antioxidants, known to neutralize toxins often associated with cancer. In addition, it's recommended that smokers eat foods that stimulate a reduction of inflammation throughout the body.

Watercress

In study after study, watercress has shown extraordinary potential in the realm of cancer prevention, asthma management, and increased airflow in and out of the lungs.[176] These benefits may arise from watercress's ability to increase the level of antioxidants in the blood and to protect against damage on a cellular level. In addition to numerous vitamins and minerals, watercress is a rich natural source of lutein and zeaxanthin.

Apples

An apple or two a day really can keep the doctor away. Apples contain a flavonoid known as khellin, which studies have shown helps reduce inflammation in the lungs, thereby improving airflow.

Citrus Fruits

Citrus fruits, including orange and grapefruit, contain vitamin C and vitamin E, powerful antioxidants that help alleviate inflammation. Grapefruit in particular is recommended given that it contains naringin, a flavonoid that blocks enzymes thought to activate cancer cells.

Avocado

The antioxidant glutathione is found in avocados. Avocado is therefore recommended along with the other antioxidants.[177] Avocado also contains vitamin E and healthy unsaturated fats, both of which are recommended for lung health of smokers. Vitamin E is depleted by nicotine and other chemicals found in cigarettes.

Spiritual Adrenaline Inspiration: **Austin C., California**

Austin C. is in recovery from alcohol and cocaine.

Getting sober is full-body recovery: mental, emotional, social, spiritual, and physical. At first, the physical seemed pretty basic. The rule was, don't drink and your body will heal itself. Getting sober from alcohol and drugs almost immediately stopped my night sweats, thudding hangover-induced headaches, nausea from bingeing, nasal congestion from snorting, and general physical malaise. In the years before I got sober, my diet grew increasingly unhealthy. In the final months, I ate only pizza slices and fast food—whatever was quick and cheap, because I couldn't afford much else.

Once I got sober, I would eat fuller meals, but I would go overboard with indulgence—huge portions of wildly unhealthy food and a pint of ice cream every night. I wasn't drinking, but physically I was not headed down the right path.

Two things happened. First, I realized I needed to take control of my eating habits. I did this by teaching myself how to cook—a barstool goal I never imagined I'd pursue. I got my hands on a how-to cookbook from a leading chef and started preparing healthy meals for myself, turning nutrition into a passion rather than a chore. As I became increasingly aware of the ingredients I was putting into my body, my nutrition choices became healthier and more sustainable.

Second, I took up running. I believed that the only way to lose weight was with a mix of diet and exercise. The gym was always such a bore and I preferred being outdoors, so I tried a Couch to 5K running program. To my shock, I found running extraordinarily enjoyable. I was accomplishing goals and distances that I never imagined. My body, freed from the ravages and fatigue of drugs and booze, was able to sustain first three miles, then my first race at 6.2 miles (10K).

Far from the unhealthy body I always assumed I had—the body I polluted with drinking—my body was becoming stronger, capable of conquering longer and longer distances. I finished a half-marathon. I stuck to running. A year later, in 2016, I finished the New York City Marathon! That accomplishment of running 26.2 miles, unimaginable to me only a few years before, was totally the result of getting sober, staying sober, and taking control of my physical being through mindful nutrition and sustained exercise.

For me, nutrition and exercise are not "outside issues." They go hand in hand with sobriety and the Twelve Steps. By doing the Twelve Steps, I have learned that to maintain mental and spiritual sobriety, I must also maintain physical sobriety. Every morning when I go out for a run, every time I cross the finish line of the many races I have now run, the rush of exhilaration I feel is a direct reminder that all of this is only possible because I got sober. This was the twelve-step promises coming to life. This was the Twelve Steps in action—free of resentments, in conscious contact with some force higher than myself, at the peak of my physical fitness, and at the age of forty-one.

My advice for those trying to incorporate exercise into recovery is to try new physical activities. Anything you may have the slightest interest in—swimming, biking, badminton, trapeze school, fencing, karate—go try it out. See what it does for you and how it makes you feel. It cannot sound like a chore. It cannot be something where you roll your eyes and march out to do it because you feel like you "should." Find an activity that sounds fun and interesting, and even the idea of it will make you feel happy.

Join a club for the activity, as I did for running. We have spent so many hours in bars or isolated in our apartments drinking that to go outside and meet other people doing healthy activities opens doors to a whole new way of living and a whole new way of connecting with other people.

CHAPTER TEN

Your Exercise Toolbox

It's time to begin to integrate conscious contact with your body into your twelve-step lifestyle. With a basic understanding of the interrelationship between your mental and physical health, you can now apply exercise tools to improve both. Joseph Pilates believed "physical fitness is the first requisite of happiness."[178] You don't start by running a marathon, competing in the Ironman Triathlon, or other all-consuming activities that take years of training and practice. You start with a walk around the block, taking the stairs instead of the elevator, and becoming comfortable engaging in activities in a group setting.

Apply Your Internal Measures
Your blood work tells the story of the internal health of your body. Depending on results, you will want to focus on the type of exercise that is most beneficial to you. Of course, it would be reckless to begin any exercise program without your doctor's guidance, especially for people with a history of long-term substance abuse.

Keep in mind that your body has an amazing capacity to heal and that exercise is a potent healing medicine. Don't let your blood work get you down or stop you from beginning the Spiritual Adrenaline program. Your body will heal as you make conscious contact with it and as you provide it with the self-care it both needs and deserves.

Apply Your External Measures

If you have a beer belly and you want to get rid of it, you have to have your waist measurement done on day one to avoid self-sabotage. Some changes you may not be able to see in the mirror can be revealed by a photo taken a week, a month, or a couple of months prior to now. You might think you look "fat" when you look in the mirror, but a scale will confirm that you lost weight. To avoid self-sabotage, make sure to have metrics against which you can accurately judge progress. Remember, it's "progress, not perfection." If you are looking to add muscle to your upper and/or lower body, you need to measure those muscles and track your progress. If you are looking to lean out your whole body, it becomes important to measure body fat and weight. Also, the type of exercise you engage in should be consistent with your overall physical goals. It makes no sense to start on day one without a plan. So make sure to set your baseline before getting started.

Match Nutrition to Exercise

In the previous chapter, I introduced you to nutritional tools, recovery superfoods, and Addiction Paleo. Now is the time to begin thinking about how to match what you are eating to your overall exercise goals. Recommended amounts of calories and macronutrients vary depending on your goal. If you are looking to add muscle, you want to increase consumption of protein and glucose. If you are looking to lean out, you want to keep protein stable and reduce glucose and other sugars, starches, and carbs. Whatever your goal, you want to keep healthy fats stable.

I provide sample detox, thirty- and ninety-day Spiritual Adrenaline lifestyle plans in Chapters Twelve to Fourteen. All of these plans are customizable to your needs and goals. Remember, what works for one person may not work for others. There is no "one size fits all" solution. You'll have to experiment until you find what works for you.

The Major Types of Exercise
Cardiovascular

This type of exercise increases your heart rate and includes activities such as a brisk walk, jogging, biking, sprinting, running, swimming, and many different types of aerobic activities and classes at the gym. If your goal is to improve your cardiovascular health, start slowly with cardiovascular exercise.

There are two major types of cardiovascular training: high-intensity interval training, known as "HIIT," and low-intensity steady-state training, known as "LISS."

HIIT means rapidly increasing heart rate for a short amount of time, followed by a rest period or continuing cardio at a much lower heart rate—in other words, fifteen seconds to a minute at your maximum heart rate and then one minute of rest or low intensity. CrossFit is a good example of HIIT training. HIIT training is efficient at burning fat and increasing metabolic rate, and can be done anywhere, as no equipment is necessary. For example, you can go to a park and sprint for thirty seconds, and then rest, then sprint again for another thirty seconds, and then rest again. I recommend HIIT for those who are in serious training to lose weight or get rid of hard-to-burn body fat, or are about to engage in an activity that requires being able to handle both HIIT and LISS aerobic levels. The best example that comes to mind is mountain climbing.

LISS training means working out at a consistent rate, about 50 percent of your maximum heart rate, for a long period of time. Good examples of LISS workouts are a long walk, a leisurely jog, or a relaxed swim or workout on a stationary bike or elliptical trainer at the gym for more than twenty minutes. I recommend LISS training for people who are new to exercise, have joint problems or other physical injuries, or are recovering from injuries. If your blood tests confirm low IGF or growth hormone, I also recommend LISS to avoid injury.

There are five zones in cardiovascular exercise that you need to be aware of. These zones are based upon the physiological effect and the corresponding effort it takes to get there. You can train with a heart-rate monitor or on equipment at the gym that tracks your heart rate. Each zone corresponds to how hard and fast your heart is working.

> **Zone 1:** The aerobic recovery zone is at 50 to 60 percent of your maximum heart rate, or MaxHR. In this zone, the body burns fat for energy and allows muscles to replenish their blood sugar. This is the easiest of the zones.

> **Zone 2:** This zone is at 70 percent of maximum heart rate, where the body is most efficient at building endurance.

Zone 3: The last aerobic zone is on the borderline with anaerobic function. It is between 70 and 80 percent of maximum heart rate. Anaerobic means your body has little or no more available glucose and looks to fat and other stores for its primary energy source to maintain activity.

Zone 4: This zone represents 80 to 90 percent of maximum heart rate. This is the anaerobic threshold zone in which your body burns fat stores.

Zone 5: This zone is at 90 to 100 percent of maximum heart rate. This is an anaerobic training zone and usually is reached in interval training or during other short bursts of maximum energy, for example, running a sprint.

Another simple way to measure your heart rate is by timing your pulse. Using the tips of two fingers (not your thumb), find the blood vessels located on the thumb side of your wrist. When you find the pulse, press for ten seconds. Count the number of pulses and multiply by six. According to the American Heart Association, here are the number of beats and estimated heart rate.

Age	50% Maximum Heart Rate	100% Maximum Heart Rate
20	100–170	200+
40	90–153	180
60	80–136	160

Weight Training

If you are looking to increase muscle mass and improve bone health and density, then weight training is for you. However, there are many more benefits to weight training. According to Arnold Schwarzenegger, "Building muscle builds you up in every part of your life. . . . As you witness the fruits of your labor, your self-worth and self-confidence improve and these traits will color your work and interpersonal relationships."[179] Weight training can be done in a number of ways. Free weights refer to dumbbells and barbells. Some of these have fixed weights while others can be adjusted. Another option is using Nautilus equipment or other machines that work out isolated muscle groups. Kettlebells are another way to lift weight. The goal with weight training, unlike with cardiovascular exercise, is to increase your body weight by adding muscle mass. Muscle mass is heavier than fat and requires more nutrients to sustain. Muscle mass also speeds up your metabolism. However, there are additional benefits to weight training.

The discipline, sacrifice, and persistence it takes to begin and follow through on your weight training self-care program will benefit you in ways that are hard to foresee at the start.

Keep this in mind if you are considering weight training as part of your self-care program: the type of training you pursue affects both the type of foods and how much you eat. If you are looking to add muscle, you must eat more—not only more, but real food. Protein powder and a poor diet just won't work. If you are looking to lean out and show your rips and cuts, you will eat less. The point is that you will vary your nutrition to help you achieve your goal. If you are adding muscle, keep in mind that you will be adding weight. If you are seeking to lose weight, be prepared to lose not just fat but also some muscle. For most people, it will be almost impossible to add muscle while losing weight.

CrossFit

Created by Glen Glassman, CrossFit is series of functional movements performed at high intensity. These workouts incorporate aspects of gymnastics, weightlifting, running, rowing, and more. Glassman refers to the movements in CrossFit as the "core movements of life." Many of the movements in CrossFit replicate motion and activities from outside a gym setting. CrossFit is probably the most effective way to get a full-body workout in the least amount of time. According to Glassman, "By employing a constantly varied approach to training, functional movements and intensity lead to dramatic gains in fitness."[180]

Other proponents of CrossFit claim that the workouts elevate growth hormone in the blood for up to twenty-four hours and that the high-intensity workout reaps benefits, like fat burning, for days afterward.[181]

I asked Todd Smith, a former heroin addict in recovery, who recently graduated from college with a degree in psychology and is now a trainer at Addict2Athlete in Colorado, what a newcomer to CrossFit needs to know. Here's what Todd had to say:

> Do not be discouraged or intimidated; measure your progress against yourself and nobody else; be humble and let go of your ego; don't be afraid to ask for help (we were all beginners once); and the more you put into your training, the better the results you will see..

Yoga

Many yoga platforms focus on individuals in the recovery community, as yoga integrates the physical, mental, and spiritual components of health. In the *Textbook of Yoga Psychology*, Ramamurti S. Mishra, MD, describes yoga this way:

> Though the mind is invisible, the mind's operations are recognized in its action and reaction on the body. All physical and physiological phenomena are manifestations of psychic phenomena. Vice versa, psychic phenomena manifest physiological phenomena. Mind and body are not separate and distinct realities.[182]

Yoga challenges us to recognize the interrelationship of your body and mind—it integrates breath, which provides fresh, oxygenated blood to your limbs and organs, and leaves regular practitioners with a sense of wholeness and union of the body, mind, and spirit.

The *Yoga Sutras of Patanjali*[183] contains the ancient teachings relating to the birth of yoga. The translation by Sri Swami Satchidananda is required reading for every student who seeks to be certified by the Yoga Alliance, the international yoga accrediting organization. The sutras speak to the physical practice of stretching for stress reduction, known as "hatha yoga." Hatha yoga was designed to "facilitate the real practice of yoga," namely, the understanding of and complete mastery over the mind. The meaning of *yoga* is "science of the mind."[184] In the context of how yoga can assist in your twelve-step recovery, the sutras give the following guidance:

> We all want to know more about our minds: how they work and how we can work with them. This field is closer to us

than anything else in life. It may be interesting and useful to know how to fix a car or cook a meal or how atoms are split. But something that holds a more immediate and vital interest for thoughtful people is their own mind. What is the mind? This is the subject matter of the ancient science of . . . yoga.[185]

The Twelve Steps include reflecting internally, assessing your motives, learning to control impulses, and readjusting your reactions to emotions as well as your thinking in order to reinforce positive lifestyle choices and deter negative choices. The wisdom of the ancients, embodied in yoga, has succeeded for thousands of years in helping those searching for a deeper personal meaning. It can be a powerful tool in your recovery as well. For anyone looking to understand the basics of a yoga practice, breath, and meditation, another helpful text is *The Heart of Yoga: Developing a Personal Practice* by T. K. V. Desikachar.[186]

Pilates

Pilates is a "unique system of stretching and strengthening exercises . . . [to] strengthen and tone muscles, improve posture, provide flexibility and balance, unite body and mind, and create a more streamlined shape."[187] Created by Joseph Pilates in the early part of the twentieth century, Pilates exercises are probably the most effective way to develop core strength. Joseph Pilates was quite sick during his youth, so he invented different exercises that helped him to overcome his childhood illnesses. Over time, he became physically strong. During World War I, he used the exercises he developed with great success on injured soldiers. The soldiers he treated had a more successful recovery from physical injury than untreated soldiers did.

Pilates focused on what he called the powerhouse, which we now call the core. The core region includes the abdomen, the serratus anterior, and the lower part of the back. These are the parts of your body that support almost all activity in both your upper and lower body. A strong core is necessary for a strong and healthy spinal cord.

When asked why he created Pilates, Joseph Pilates said he believed that "in order to achieve happiness it is imperative to gain mastery of your body."[188] He explained that "only through balance of the physical, mental, and spiritual" could the ideal lifestyle be attained. "Through visualization, physical strengthening, and stretching of the body, mental vigor and improved blood flow returns to inactive brain cells. This renewed spirit of thought and movement is the first step toward stress reduction, grace of movement, alacrity, and a greater enjoyment of life."

Joseph Pilates based his program on nine principles. These principles will resonate with anyone in recovery.

1. *Concentration:* Concentration is a key element to connect the body and mind. In order to work on your body, Pilates argued that you "must be present with your mind."[189] He taught students to focus on the muscle they are working out and notice how the muscle moves and the body responds. By focusing on the muscle, you can feel the area working. He described that as the "power of the mind."[190]

2. *Control:* Pilates taught students to control their muscle movements. Sloppy, inappropriate movement leads to injuries, so he taught students to stay in the present and control every muscle movement.

3. *Center:* A strong core is necessary, as all energy radiates from the core to the limbs and the outer extremities of the body.

4. *Fluidity:* Fluidity is prioritizing the "grace of motion" over the speed with which the motion is undertaken.

5. *Precision:* This includes doing fewer movements and focusing on getting it right as opposed to many half-hearted or careless movements.

6. *Breath:* Employing full inhalations and exhalations to expel stale air and noxious gases from deep within the lungs, one can replenish fresh air in the lungs, which then travels via the blood to revitalize the body.

7. *Imagination:* Pilates believed our mind acts as a switchboard through which we can signal instinctive physical responses; therefore, creative thought enhances our movements.

8. *Intuition:* Intuition means listening to your body and making decisions that are consistent with what your body is telling you. For example, if your shoulder hurts, let it rest; don't just continue to work it out. Pilates believed that most people take their instinct

and intuition for granted. Pay attention to the signs and signals your body sends you.

9. *Integration:* Integration involves the ability to see your body as an integrated whole. Pilates did not believe in isolating one muscle group; rather, he recommended working out the entire body through exercises all originating in the core yet integrating all muscle groups. Pilates strongly cautioned against isolating muscles; he taught that this would cause imbalance to the body and ultimately cause injury to joints and other damage.

Recovery-Specific Exercise Programs

Y12SR: Yoga of Twelve-Step Recovery

Nikki Myers created Yoga of Twelve-Step Recovery, or Y12SR, in order to integrate the benefits of a traditional yoga practice with the benefits of a traditional twelve-step practice. Myers says, "The issues live in our tissues. Y12SR connects the dots between the ancient wisdom of yoga, the practical tools of twelve-step programs, and the latest research on trauma healing and neurobiology. As part of a holistic recovery program, it works in tandem with traditional treatment to address the physical, mental, and spiritual disease of addiction."[191]

Y12SR is designed to serve a wide spectrum of people recovering from "all manifestations of addiction, from behavioral addictions to substance abuse—creating a safe place on the mat where trauma can be released." Individuals can attend trainings and become certified to facilitate Y12SR meetings in their local communities. Meetings are currently available in community settings across the United States and in other countries. Given the success of the program, Y12SR is being offered as a therapy option in a growing number of addiction-recovery treatment centers.

Yoga of Recovery

Yoga of Recovery is a retreat-based program integrating the wisdom of yoga and Ayurveda with the tools of twelve-step recovery. It is open to all who are looking to overcome self-destructive or addictive tendencies. The program quotes the Big Book when it describes sobriety/abstinence as a "daily reprieve contingent on the maintenance of our spiritual condition."

This combination of yoga, Ayurveda, and the tools of twelve-step recovery offers a unique recovery approach. What distinguishes Yoga of Recovery from other recovery-based programs is the integration of Ayurveda, the medical/holistic healing practice and sister science of yoga. Ayurveda is the traditional Hindu system of medicine that aims to balance body systems using diet, herbal treatment, and yogic breathing.

IntenSati

IntenSati, created by and taught by Patricia Moreno, is an innovative and original format for integrating body and mind. I describe the IntenSati Method as a cross between kickboxing and yoga, done while yelling positive affirmations such as "I am beautiful!" and "No more fear!" Moreno describes her program as a "unique, holistic approach to dieting and fitness. IntenSati will teach you how to use your conscious, goal-making mind to access and awaken your spiritual or subconscious mind."[192, 193]

IntenSati has grown into a worldwide phenomenon. Today, Moreno holds conferences with inspirational speakers and retreats in the United States and abroad, and has developed numerous leadership-training programs that are innovative and consistent with a twelve-step approach to recovery.

Sober Active Communities

The Phoenix

Scott Strode is in long-term recovery from alcohol and cocaine. I consider Scott the "founding father" of the "active sober" movement. Scott was the first to organize a sober community of people interested in integrating nutrition and exercise into their recovery. In his recovery, Scott began to train hard and compete in Ironman competitions. He also began to climb mountains. Scott shared on how these physical challenges helped him grow: "Every time I finish a race or reach the summit, I thought of myself as less of an addict and more of an athlete." To pursue his new passion for hiking and climbing, Scott relocated from Boston to Denver.

In 2006, he and some friends founded Phoenix Multisport in Boulder, Colorado. The organization is now known as The Phoenix. The organization does not integrate the Twelve Steps or recommend any other specific recovery model. Rather, it promotes a healthy and active environment revolving around exercise and community. When I asked Scott to explain why he created The Phoenix, he told me, "It broke my heart to see people come out of treatment and not have an active community." He continued, "Competing in the Ironman and other sports helped me to find myself. Through Phoenix, I can show someone I believe in them, oftentimes before they even believe in themselves."

At The Phoenix, people recovering from substance use disorder and anyone else who chooses to live a recovery-oriented life can come to train in a gym setting and enhance their twelve-step program. The program's only requirement is that members have "forty-eight hours of sobriety and follow a simple code of conduct. With this forty-eight hour requirement if a person relapses, they more likely to return to our sober active community."

The types of physical activity at Phoenix include climbing, hiking, running, CrossFit strength training, yoga, and road and mountain biking, as well as social events that help build a sense of community. The group has an annual trip to Moab, Utah, for a weekend of hiking, camping, and active fellowship. The program has expanded beyond Boulder and presently offers programs in numerous cities in Colorado (Boulder, Denver, Colorado Springs, Westminster, Wheatridge); Boston, Massachusetts; Orange County, California; Portland, Maine; Portsmouth, New Hampshire (summer surf); Boise, Idaho; Billings, Montana; Philadelphia, Pennsylvania; Atlanta, Georgia; Tampa Bay, Florida; and Dallas, Texas.

The organization's goal is simple and makes common sense: "to expand people's sober community while creating a safe environment. People choosing to live a sober lifestyle often find it necessary to make changes to many aspects of their lives, including their social circles, in order to maintain sobriety. Abrupt changes in lifestyle can lead to loss of support networks and often cause people to become isolated."[194] Scott and the Phoenix have now worked with tens of thousands of people in recovery, and the number continues to grow.

To track progress toward its mission, The Phoenix collects surveys from its members after three month of participating in its programs. In December of 2017, The Phoenix issued its findings in an Impact Report. The report measured the program's success rates in achieving short-term sobriety and changes in attitudes about recovery.[195] Data was collected from 241 active Phoenix participants from program sites around the country. Participants were asked to share their impression about recovery and how their view changed, if at all, over a three-month period. The results confirmed what Scott and other staff at The Phoenix had known all along from working with people firsthand. Over the three months, 91 percent reported having more favorable attitudes about sober activities; 85 percent reported increased self-efficacy; 81 percent reported they were better able to cope with stress; 76 percent reported improved self-esteem; and 81 percent reported feeling a greater sense of purpose in life. The dramatic increase in positive self-image and growth reflected in the Impact Report is consistent with findings of other peer-reviewed studies.

However, the Impact Report contains some more good news regarding fitness and overall health: 71 percent confirmed a greater motivation to remain sober; 71 percent reported improved overall health; 67 percent reported improved physical health; and 76 percent reported improved mental health. Three-quarters of the original 241 participants, or 75 percent, remained sober over the three months, and of the 25 percent who relapsed, 66 percent said that participation in the Phoenix program was the major reason they returned later to sobriety.

Phoenix has also supported other local active sober organizations including providing small start-up donations or other support.

Addict2Athlete

Recovering methamphetamine addict Rob Archuleta and his wife Sheena Archuleta, a recovering crack addict, founded Addict2Athlete (A2A) in April of 2009 in Pueblo, Colorado. The group began as a running club that ran for a half-hour and then attended a half-hour meeting. Originally housed at a martial arts dojo, the group now meets at Stay Invincible CrossFit in Pueblo. Since getting into recovery, Rob has become an Ironman triathlete and marathon runner. He has also become a certified personal trainer, CrossFit level 1 trainer, and certified Insanity workout instructor. He has also been certified as a chemical abuse counselor and prevention specialist.

Rob's experience as a person in recovery with exercise training has made him a leader in the integration of recovery and exercise science. Rob shared his belief on how to succeed in recovery: "Recovery philosophies are wonderful, but when the mind and the body are not in sync, the war on addiction is more difficult. Having seen the need for the mind and the body to be as one, Addict2Athlete was born."

What makes the A2A program unique is that it's not step based and does not follow the disease model of addiction recovery. Rather, A2A offers its own cutting-edge curriculum developed by Rob and Sheena to help those in recovery overcome antisocial behavior and develop positive life skills. The goal of the curriculum is to assist members of the recovery community to reintegrate into society by relearning basic life skills such as healthy eating, positive relationships, and self-care for both the body and mind.

Here's a look at the topics covered over the eight-week program: Criminal History/Low Self-Control; Antisocial Attitude/Orientation; Antisocial Companions; Antisocial Personality Pattern; Dysfunctional Family/Marriage/Relationship; Education and Employment; Leisure and Recreation; and Alcohol/Drug Problems. Notably, the final week focuses on alcohol and other drugs, with the first seven focused on "outside issues." I asked Rob to describe A2A's philosophy. Here's what he had to say:

> Recovery is not about being sober; it is about recovering aspects of our lives that we lost in addiction. What have you lost? Respect, trust, employment? If those aspects of your life are not improving, then you are not in recovery. You are probably a sober a##hole. Remember, sobriety is not the absence of desire, but the desire for something greater. I desire drugs and women all the time; I just desire my life and my wife more!! Sobriety is like marriage. The priest asked, "Do you forsake all others?" I said yes!!!! He didn't ask, "Do you promise not to desire others?" If he had asked that I would have been lying!
>
> Make a commitment to recovery, find something you desire more than drugs, and grab onto it as tight as you can. I once created an acronym for DESIRE: Don't Expect Serenity It's Really Earned. Serenity is earned with every mile you run, every plate of food you push away, and every meeting you attend. Work for recovery, work the same way you did when you were looking for drugs.

A2A, now in both Colorado and New Mexico, is growing and will likely expand to numerous other cities and states in the next few years. A2A serves mainstream recovery clients and those who are referred to A2A by the court system as a condition of probation. With regard to ex-offenders, the success of the A2A program was evaluated over a two-year period by the 10th Judicial District, Department of Probation, in Pueblo, Colorado.[196] The evaluation came to the following key findings: A2A participants on parole were "significantly less likely" to violate parole; the A2A program benefited both "male and female participants and . . . probation clients from different race/ethnic groups"; and "graduates of the A2A program demonstrated improvements in four indices of physical fitness. Fitness activities provide probation clients with positive focus for their time and energy. . . . [T]ime spent at the gym may replace time spent alone or with antisocial peers, reducing the time and opportunity for recidivating."[197]

ROCovery Fitness

Yana Khashper and Sean Smith, two of the cofounders of ROCovery Fitness in Rochester, New York, describe the program as a "supportive community of physically active individuals brought together by sober living, committed to creating an environment of healing and recovery." The goal of ROCovery is to empower "members, friends, and families . . . to discover their inner strength and confidence through adventure, fun, and camaraderie."[198] In May of 2017, ROCovery opened the first active sober-living center in New York state. Among the activities sponsored by ROCovery include candlelight vinyasa yoga, boot camp at local parks on weekend mornings, a gym in its community center, and hikes in the parks and mountains surrounding Rochester.

All of this began when a group of people decided to put together a hike as a positive, healthy activity for people in the addiction recovery community. About a dozen people joined the group's founders Yana Khashper and Sean Smith for that first hike. Reflecting on how the group got started, Yana said, "We were looking for an alternative to relapse. We thought that maybe fitness could be the piece we were missing in our recovery." ROCovery Fitness has over 1,000 individuals who have participated in adventures, activities, and community events that the group sponsors.

For the future, ROCovery is focused on "providing a safe fitness-oriented community for individuals recovering from addiction . . . while fostering a commitment to change by replacing maladaptive patterns of living through the connectedness of like-minded individuals pursuing wellness, fitness, and outdoor living."

Recovery 2.0

If you are looking for others interested in a healthy recovery lifestyle, *Recovery 2.0: Move Beyond Addiction and Upgrade Your Life* by Tommy Rosen is a best-selling book and online platform.[199] According to Tommy's website, the community "numbers approximately 250,000 globally and consists mostly of people whose lives have been touched by addiction in one form or another. Some are dealing with active addiction. Others are on a path of recovery. Many of us are family members or loved ones of a person dealing with addiction. And still others work in the recovery field." In addition to Rosen's book and website, Recovery 2.0 holds internet-based conferences featuring a wide assortment of leading thinkers in the recovery field, coaching programs, and intensive retreats.

Exercise Tools

Integrate Your Twelve-Step Practice with Exercise

If you don't live near one of these local organizations, you can join their online communities or create your own by timing your workouts around your twelve-step practice. For example, park ten blocks away from your meeting and walk there. Bike to a meeting instead of driving. If your gym is near where you attend meetings, then work out before or after and share about it at your twelve-step meeting. By sharing about how exercise makes you feel and about your efforts to integrate a healthy lifestyle into your recovery, you make it easier to meet healthy and sober people who will support your efforts.

"Bookend" Your Twelve-Step Practice with Exercise

Another powerful way to integrate exercise into your twelve-step program is to bookend your workout with your daily meeting. To bookend, plan a morning meeting and then an evening exercise program, or vice versa. This way you begin your day in a positive mind-set and end it in a positive mind-set. Follow my nutritional recommendations during the day, and your energy should come from protein and healthy fat sources rather than caffeine and sugar. This will help you avoid spiking your blood sugar, lessen mood swings and cravings, and keep you in a positive frame of mind throughout the day between your meeting and workout.

Exercise in Nature

Combining exercise with the outdoors delivers twice as much punch as a workout at the gym. Who wants to be inside on a beautiful day? For many, connecting with nature is necessary to feel a spiritual connection with their higher power. Certainly for me, running or biking on concrete in the city lacks the appeal of climbing a mountain, getting out on the water, and just being away from other human beings to enjoy solitude or the company of friends who also enjoy living off the grid. Studies have proven that people who exercise in a green or natural setting derive greater psychological benefits than those who work out indoors do.[200] "Short-term exposure [even five minutes] to outdoor exercise improves both self-esteem and mood irrespective of duration, intensity, location, gender, age, and health status."[201] This is especially true for people suffering from depression.

There are so many activities that enable you to exercise in nature: for example, paddleboarding, kiteboarding, windsurfing, surfing, walking, long-distance cycling, mountain biking, skating, Rollerblading, skateboarding, and hiking.

Turn Your Workout into a Meditation

It's easy to turn your workout, whether cardio or strength training, into an active meditation. If you are planning to do some cardio, focus on your breath as your heart rate increases. For example, on your exhale, focus on your character defects and exhale them out. Go through your Sixth Step in your mind and exhale those defects right out. It's a great way to let go of the baggage you need to toss to lighten your load in recovery. On the inhale, bring in loving kindness, empathy, and gratitude for your life, health, and recovery.

This type of meditation can be done with or without music. There are plenty of meditation apps and programs available to download. I prefer to create my own meditations, but you may like someone else's guided meditations.

If you are weight training, you can follow the "breathe in, breathe out" meditation on defects or you can modify it to fit your personal situation. When weight training, you are doing multiple reps of each muscle group. The repetition of weight training makes it the perfect complement to meditation. Here's another meditation you can do while working out. On the inhale, breathe in good intentions toward someone you owe amends to. On the exhale, breathe out the resentment or guilt you have toward that person. By focusing the mind and breath on discharging the negative and taking in the good through breath, hopefully you will feel lighter—like you've dropped the rock or otherwise lightened your load in sobriety. This way, you turn your self-care program into a physical and spiritual workout.

For either of these examples, to the extent possible, notice your muscles at work. Notice your veins and the blood flowing through them. Your body is a remarkable gift that you abused and took for granted. If you are healthy enough to work out, appreciate the gift. The very act of working out is a self-care amends. Reflect on how much you will be able to accomplish with a healthy body in recovery. Marvel at how your body survived the abuse you inflicted on it while using. Contemplate how different things will be if you stick to your self-care program.

Nutrient Timing

If you are looking to build muscle, it's important to time your meal to be almost immediately after your weight-training workout. The half-hour after working out is the optimal time to get nutrients to your muscles to add mass. You will want to make sure to combine protein, carbohydrates, and BCAAs to maximize muscle growth.

If you are looking to lean out and lose fat, your meal timing will be different. To burn off calories and macronutrients, you will want to eat one hour or at least a half-hour before your workout. This way, the nutrients are in you prior to your workout and you have fuel for your workout and continue to burn it for two to three hours afterward.

If you are more experienced at working out, in order to maximize your burn, you can avoid eating after working out. This forces your body to burn existing fat stores. This is an extreme training technique and it is not recommended for beginners. It is also not healthy if practiced over the long term.

Over Forty? Twice a Day

If you are over forty, you will want to try to work out twice a day—your main workout in the morning and a second and much shorter cardio-only set in the afternoon. The afternoon session is intended to be brief, only fifteen or twenty minutes. You need not return to the gym if you belong to one. The afternoon session can be a bike ride, vigorous walk, or jog. This reactivates your metabolism and keeps it churning.

After forty, your metabolic rate slows dramatically. The brief afternoon session will dramatically increase the results you see in a shorter period of time by keeping your metabolism churning later in the day and while you sleep. The trick with the second workout is to continue with your cardio until you feel a chill run through your body. This chill indicates that your body has burned through available glucose and is now transitioning to fat for energy. If you continue past this threshold, you will be burning excess fat and have the confidence that you are leaning out and working off excess carbs before going to bed. In most adults, this occurs at somewhere around twenty minutes of consistent mid-range cardio Zones 3 or 4. These are the zones (mentioned earlier) in which most people transition from aerobic to anaerobic or from burning available glucose to burning stored fat.

Use Technology

By using technology, you can unshackle yourself from your home, computer, or desk. Rather than having life revolve around work, you can modify things and have life revolve around your health and self-care program. This is a radically different way to think and live, made possible because of technology.

Let me share with you part of my workout routine by way of example. In my morning cardio session, I bring my iPad. While riding the bike, I check all my emails and respond. I check Facebook and my bank balance (not to check how rich I am but to reconfirm that I am usually broke and need to work to pay my bills). I journal, start my food log, and go over my calendar to prioritize my day and schedule for the days ahead. I do all of this while burning fat and churning up my metabolism for the next six to eight hours. I am accomplishing multiple responsibilities all at once. When I concentrate on these things while riding, fifteen minutes, thirty-five minutes, or even an hour can pass unbelievably quickly. I get a tremendous sense of satisfaction that I am working and engaging in my twelve-step program at the same time.

In the afternoon, I often bring drafts of documents to proof or go through my mail during my cardio session. I also keep up with my food log and journals and use the afternoon session to write about how my day went, what areas I need to work on, and what I am grateful for. In 2013, I took an advanced-level nutrition course streaming on my iPad while riding the bike at the gym. I often treat myself to leisure reading in my afternoon session. For me, this means recovery-oriented books and books on Buddhism or nutrition. It's great to interrupt the day with some afternoon me-time to reconnect with my higher power.

Once you get into the discipline of getting to the gym and putting cardio time to such productive use, you won't mind doing cardio, and soon enough larger amounts of time won't seem like such a big deal. You will not be focused on how long you've been going but rather on how productive you have been.

Fitbit and Your Exercise Program

A study released in September of 2017 researched the impact of technology-supported workouts on the relapse rates of women in recovery who also suffered from depression.[202] The women participating had their exercise tracked by a Fitbit, which is a wireless activity tracker that you wear, usually around your wrist, to track heart rate, steps, and other data during your workouts. In this study, the Fitbit captured three measures: number of steps, minutes of physical activity, and the number of times during the twelve-week study the participants actually worked out.[203] The study found that the women who regularly participated in exercise and who tracked their workouts had a lower rate of relapse than women who either failed to regularly engage in exercise or who simply chose not to exercise at all. Another conclusion of the study was that women who tracked the number of steps and total minutes of exercise seemed to structure their exercise and progressively increase both the number of steps and total minutes exercised over the twelve-week period. Overall, there was a total 72 percent increase in steps per day over the twelve weeks.[204] Another intriguing conclusion was that physical activity was "significantly correlated with reductions in levels of depression and anxiety in participants." Research seems to confirm a direct correlation between tracking exercise in a structured way over time—that is, tracking steps, minutes, and number of sessions—and lower relapse rates, depression, and anxiety. If Fitbit doesn't work for you, check out some other technology to help your workouts in recovery.

Cardio Lift

If you are not ready to get on the bike, elliptical, or treadmill, I recommend you try what I call cardio lift. Cardio lift means utilizing free weights and Nautilus machines with minimal or no rest between machines by combining body parts worked. To cardio lift, you've got to get to the gym early, when it's slow in the afternoon, or around closing time. You will need the gym crowd to be light since you simply cannot cardio lift in a crowded gym.

I cardio lift every day during my morning workout. Cardio lift permits you to work through your routine at a more rapid pace, maximizing your heart rate. You will want to try to get your heart rate to at least Zone 3 and, if possible, Zone 4 for brief periods. This enables you to build muscle while burning fat and working out multiple muscle groups at the same time.

I usually break up my cardio lift routine by alternating abs, obliques, or serratus exercises with upper body, core, or leg routines. The obliques and serratus are muscles that run along the sides of your chest and are often ignored in favor of the six-pack muscles of your belly. By working the obliques and serratus, you strengthen your core, which helps enhance your six-pack. You also enhance overall core strength and support for your upper body. Women get particular benefit from strengthening these muscles, as osteoporosis is often prevalent in postmenopausal women and muscle strength and bone health are closely related.[205] The chart below gives you an idea of my three-days-on/one-day-off cardio-lift routine. Given that rest is critical, I work out three days in a row and often follow this rotation:

- **Day 1:** Pecs, abs, calves (working out pecs or chest, then abs, then calves without rest to keep heart rate elevated in a target zone)
- **Day 2:** Biceps, triceps, obliques, serratus anterior (working out arm muscles and midsection without rest to keep heart rate elevated in a target zone)

- **Day 3:** Lower back, abs, calves, legs (combining lower back, legs, and midsection workout without rest to keep heart rate elevated in a target zone)
- **Day 4:** Rest. Rest is critical for your body to avoid injury and maximize gains. By resting, you permit your body to revitalize and grow. I like to do a yoga class or light swim on my rest days.
- **Day 5:** Lats, abs, lower back (combining your lower back and midsection in a core-focused exercise)
- **Day 6:** Shoulders, abs, obliques, serratus anterior (combining upper body and midsection workout without rest to keep heart rate elevated in a target zone)
- **Day 7:** Upper back, abs, legs (combining upper body and midsection workout without rest to keep heart rate elevated in a target zone)
- **Day 8:** Rest.

By cardio lifting, you will effectively manage your time at the gym with a plan that will move your workouts along. You will have more time for living, and by being focused you will get better results in a shorter amount of time while at the gym.

There are plenty of apps you can download to help you develop your own routines beyond what I include in this book. I recommend Fitocracy, My Fitness Pal, and Daily Burn.

Basic Exercise/Nutrition Math

Here are some helpful formulas that will assist you in setting the proper intake of calories and macronutrients (proteins, carbs, fat, sugar) on a daily basis to accomplish your fitness goals. The simple way to estimate your necessary calorie intake is to simply add a zero to your weight. That takes all the nuancing out of the process and gives you a rough estimate of the range of total calories you should be taking in on any given day. If you think I'm wrong, try the more complicated methods and then see if I'm far off or not. (The "add a zero" method does not work for those in serious training for competitions, triathlons, marathons, and so on. If you are in serious training, you need to consult with a sports nutritionist or someone else who can guide you on how many calories you will need to expend.)

Here are some general guidelines:[206]

Men	
If your body fat is:	You should eat this many calories:
28 percent and higher	2,300–3,500
20–27 percent	2,200–3,000
13–19 percent	1,800–2,800
12 percent and under	1,000–1,800
Women	
37 percent and higher	1,700–2,200
30–36 percent	1,600–1,850
23–29 percent	1,400–1,750
22 percent and under	1,250–2,000

If you are following the Addiction Paleo program, I recommend consuming most of your carbs from the time you wake up until 3:00 p.m. and then cutting them off until bedtime. From 2:00 or 3:00 p.m. to bedtime, increase protein and fat and try to avoid carbs entirely. If you are counting calories and your macronutrients, I recommend that protein should compose 20 to 30 percent, healthy fats 50 to 60 percent, and carbs the remaining 20 to 30 percent. The absolute highest your carbohydrate intake should go is 30 percent.

If you are looking to maintain your muscle mass, one gram of protein per pound is sufficient. If you are looking to increase muscle mass, 2–2.5 grams is the proper range for most.

Develop a Health-Based Community

Long-term change requires us to enjoy our new activities and lifestyle. This means building healthy new relationships and a sense of community. It's critical to replace the isolation of your using days with a new routine of interacting with healthy-minded people who have a positive outlook on life. Misery loves company, but let someone else provide the company, not you. You are not in this to survive; you are reading this book because you want to *thrive*.

The internet and social media make it easy to tune into a community of like-minded people quickly. Join email lists for fitness and nutrition websites that offer suggestions on healthy exercise programs and food choices. I recommend www.bodybuilding.com, which is full of helpful information for people at all levels of fitness. If you take classes at your gym on a regular basis, you can develop healthy relationships with the staff and trainers there.

Set Realistic and Achievable Goals

Set realistic goals that are achievable and end the vicious cycle of self-sabotage caused by setting yourself up to fail. I am constantly reminding myself that life is not a sprint but a marathon. Even though I'm heading to my eighth year in my recovery from alcohol and other drugs (sixth year from nicotine), I am constantly telling myself to slow down. This is why it's important to know the results of your blood work and medical exams and what you are capable of. After years of abuse, does your body still produce the hormones necessary to engage in athletic activity? Is your body producing enough growth hormone to repair and rebuild muscle? What are your testosterone and estrogen levels like? What's your red blood cell count, and can your blood get oxygen to your organs and body when you're working out?

If your counts are low, it's not a problem. You can work with your doctor and/or personal trainer to figure out a plan. For example, if you're looking to boost your testosterone levels, focus on more-intense leg lifts and exercises. The legs contain the largest muscles in male and female bodies, and by working leg muscles intensely you stimulate your testosterone levels. There are lots of simple tricks like this to supplement what your doctor recommends.

In the short term, you can work with your doctor to supplement the vitamins, minerals, and other nutrients you take that will help you bridge from nutritionally deficient in active addiction to healthy to well-nourished in recovery. In time, your levels should stabilize. Research confirms that levels of critical hormones and blood elements, even in long-term substance abusers, return to normal after about six months of abstinence for about two thirds of people. The remaining third will need to consult their doctor and may require long-term planning. If you keep going, slowly your suffering will give way to a sense of wellness.

Increase Testosterone Naturally

Studies confirm that by working out early in the morning, you boost production of testosterone in the afternoon. Testosterone helps build and maintain muscle and is important for both men and women, although in women in lower amounts. It is undisputed that testosterone levels are highest in the morning when we first wake up and that they drop throughout the day. In a recent study, a semipro rugby team in England had their testosterone levels measured in the morning and then again in the afternoon for a period of a month. The researchers then split the team into three groups. The first group was told not to work out in the morning, the second ran five 40-meter sprints, and the third performed multiple repetitions of bench presses and squats, ran a 40-meter sprint, and then did jumping jacks. The results showed that the lifters had the highest level of afternoon testosterone, followed by the sprinters, and then the control group who did nothing.

Male and Female Biology

There's no dispute that the female body behaves differently than the male body in the context of addiction to alcohol and other drugs. Research confirmed long ago that it takes less of whatever substance is being abused and less time for women to become dependent on alcohol or their drug of choice. Science has explained the role of estrogen, a hormone produced in much larger quantities in women than in men, which impacts the dopamine reward pathway. A 2014 study concluded that estrogen impacts the neural systems that control positive and negative reinforcement, prompting the release of endorphins.[207] Because of the high level of estrogen, smaller amounts of alcohol or other drugs are needed for females to prompt the release of a larger number of endorphins than in males equivalent by body weight.

Let's look at how alcohol and a few commonly abused substances impact men and women differently.

Opioids

Women are more likely to be prescribed opioids than men and to continue to use them in the long term. Women also have an increased risk of opioid misuse related to emotional issues while men tend to abuse opioids because of legal or behavioral problems.[208]

Alcohol

Alcohol kills double the number of women than opioids do, according to CDC statistics. For example, in 2010, alcohol was responsible for the deaths of 26,000 women while 13,000 died from opioid overdose. Women develop dependence on alcohol faster than men and also develop organ damage to the liver and brain at a faster rate than men. The reason the female body is more vulnerable to alcohol dependence and damage is due to two major factors. First, women tend to weigh less than men and their bodies retain less water and more fatty tissue (for reproductive purposes) than men. Fat retains alcohol while water dilutes it. The additional fat retention in women leads to a greater likelihood of organ damage. Second, women have lower levels of alcohol dehydrogenase, an enzyme that helps to metabolize alcohol, leading to faster absorption in the bloodstream.

Nicotine

According to a Harvard University study, female smokers are more likely to have a heart attack or develop lung cancer than their male counterparts.

Respect Gender Differences

It's important to understand that male and female bodies are different and the results that can be achieved by a man may not be achievable by a woman. For example, the male body produces far more testosterone than the female body does, enabling men to add substantially more muscle.

Men also shed fat much more easily than women do. The reason is that nature designed women so they could get pregnant and reproduce. For hundreds of thousands of years, our ancestors were hunter-gatherers who ate when they could find food. Only recently have humans had such easy access to food all year round. The female anatomy, designed around preserving the species, makes it harder to shed fat.

In twelve-step programs, it is suggested that you accept the things you cannot change. So please avoid sabotaging yourself by not taking into account your gender, biology, and the natural order of things. What I am saying may not be politically correct, but it is scientifically accurate. That's what is important for those who are serious about restoring their body to health.

Rise & Grind, Reno, Nevada

Breaking from the one-size-fits-all model of many rehabilitation facilities, some recovery innovators have put their own common sense and intuition to good use and developed treatment plans geared toward women and their specific needs. Rise & Grind, a program based in Reno, Nevada, is an innovative program founded by Grant Denton. Grant overcame addiction and founded the program because he recognized the importance of exercise to recovery. Rise & Grind partnered with Life Changes, a local sober-living facility for women. Women from Life Changes who successfully complete the Rise & Grind program are given a free one-year membership to American Iron Gym, located in Reno.[209]

I asked Grant to share the top benefits of Rise & Grind for their clients.

- **The Magic 60**

  "When a woman gets into recovery she will commonly put on a significant amount of weight within the first couple of months. We call it 'the magic 60,' referring to pounds. When men in recovery put on the same sixty pounds, they often wear it with pride. However, women wear it with shame and start to miss the days when they were thinner. Unfortunately, usually when they were thinner they were using, often not eating, dehydrated, and malnourished. A lot of women in recovery will relapse to avoid being 'fat.' Exercise and proper nutrition can help them avoid this type of self-sabotage and stinking thinking."

- **Confidence**

  "When a woman is in active addiction, whether on the streets or not, she is often made to feel less than by the people she surrounds herself with. Consistent exercise and proper motivation build confidence."

- **Trust/Safety**

  "In the world of recovery, too often women are looked at as objects and, sadly, treated as such. They are often preyed upon by men and even other women. Rise & Grind is set up to make our participants feel safe. They are in a supportive and healthy environment at all times, and are surrounded by our staff who are always positive and uplifting."

- **Peer Support**

"One of the primary components of recovery is hope—hope that they can achieve what may have once seemed impossible. We offer hope by having peers for trainers, that is, someone who has lived the experience of addiction or mental illness and who can answer questions. We tie in what we learn in the gym to life lessons and help them to translate it into real-life application."[210]

Spiritual Adrenaline Inspiration: **Clayton Y., Texas**

Clayton Y. is a bodybuilder who competes in the National Physique Conference (NPC). He is also a person in long-term recovery from alcohol and cocaine abuse.

> Exercise and nutrition gave me hope when I had none, and they gave me a better sense of self-worth. When I was out control in active addiction, it felt as if I had almost no choice about what to do with my life. The drugs were in control. In recovery, I stepped into the gym and made a choice to try to take back my life. Exercise was a light in the midst of all the darkness. Good nutrition gave me the energy and propelled me to consciously awaken my spirit. Both went hand in hand as a physical and emotional cleanse. I slowly began to realize that every day in the gym, every bit of food, every choice mattered. It was like a mountain in front of me that I had to start climbing, and instead of becoming weak from the fight, I became stronger. I made the choice to become better each day.
>
> I've learned that nutrition has directly helped me in being able to cope. Consuming the right foods absolutely can bring my energy up. When I ate crappy foods, it made me feel lethargic. As a competitive bodybuilder in the NPC, I've learned how using

quality carbohydrates for energy gets my motor going in the morning and powers me through the day. Healthy fats affect my brain in how it functions and my overall health and behavior. Good nutrition helps me win the internal battle.

Exercise is my release and coping mechanism. I go to the gym and I forget every single problem. My blood circulates and my heart starts pumping hard. I've found I lose myself in this healthy addiction. I am constantly finding ways to challenge myself physically. I'm now addicted to becoming the best version of me.

My slogan is "Just Start!" First you start, then you continue, then you don't stop. There's never a finish line when you have addiction. Don't wait for when you feel like doing something. You may never feel like doing it. Force yourself to do positive things. Start exercising and taking your nutrition seriously. Believe in yourself and also surround yourself with people who believe in you and love you and reinforce healthy habits. There's lots of support out there in the fitness community. Use it. Don't run away from change. Run to it head-on!

CHAPTER ELEVEN

Your Spiritual Toolbox

In the Big Book of Alcoholics Anonymous, Bill W. wrote: "The spiritual life is not a theory. We have to live it."[211] But how exactly do we "live it"? For people who have lived in the chaos and confusion of active addiction, living spiritually sounds like a lot to ask. What does living spiritually mean? How do we get to that place? Does living spiritually mean you have to live like a monk or nun? Will you be bored? Are your days of enjoying life and having fun over?

These are critical questions, and the answers can seem elusive. Many people speak of "tools," but what exactly does that mean? You can read books, attend Eleventh Step meetings and seminars, and still have difficulty with the concept. Some tools may work for you and others not so much. Unlike nutritional and exercise tools that are fixed in science, spiritual tools are subjective. What works for one person may not work for another. So in the context of spiritual tools, each of us has to take his or her own journey until we find what works for us as an individual. If you are having difficulty with the concept, you are not alone. Many of us in recovery struggle with this topic. The key is to keep going until you find the tools that work for *you*.

In *The Tools: 5 Tools to Help You Find Courage, Creativity, and Willpower—and Inspire You to Live Life in Forward Motion* by Phil Stutz and Barry Michels,[212] the authors describe tools as mechanisms to turn problems into opportunities.[213] In many respects, the approach the authors take is similar to that of the Twelve Steps and Buddhism: you change your world when you change your perception of it. Tools can change the way you perceive the challenges you face and help you adapt from seeing yourself as a victim to "experience[ing] a level of creativity [you've] never felt before."[214] Moreover, after you've used the tools for an extended period of time, the benefits are a "daily connection to life-changing higher forces"[215] that can be like a "gift from somewhere else [that] carried an extraordinary power."

I like tools of practical application, that is, very specific acts that you can do whenever you feel like it. Rather than concepts or theories, my spiritual toolbox focuses on tools that require action. Once the action is taken, the consequence should become apparent. If you work the tools that follow, the consequence may not be what you expected, but it will be positive.

Airplane Mode

The greatest impediment to your spiritual health these days is technology. "This rapidly progressing world with its ever-increasing faster tempo of living demands that we be physically fit and alert in order that we may succeed in the unceasing race with keen competition, which rewards the 'go-getter' but bypasses the 'no-getter.'"[216] Sounds like something someone may have said yesterday or today, but it's actually a quote from Joseph Pilates in 1945. If the tempo was too much for the average human in 1945, think about the stressors we are under today.

Quite frankly, the demands are overwhelming. Human beings were not designed to live in the manner in which most of us do today. Our instinct and primal nature are to hunt and gather food. The lack of physical activity is counterinstinctual. Also, the constant bombardment with electronic stimuli can overwhelm anyone. To cover up the stress and anxiety, many people drink alcohol or take prescription and/or illicit drugs. It's incredibly difficult to practice mindfulness, because we are always connected via wireless and the internet to other people, places, and things. We are somewhere else mentally when texting, emailing, calling, or surfing the web.

Increasingly, researchers are confirming that electronic devices are addictive not by accident, but by design. Adam Alter studied the topic at length for his book *Irresistible: The Rise of Addictive Technology and the Business of Keeping Us Hooked.*[217] His fascinating exposé begins by disclosing that Steve Jobs, the man who brought the world the iPad, would not allow his own children to use it.[218] In a 2010 interview with the *New York Times,* Jobs said, "We limit how much technology our kids use." But Jobs was not alone. Other Silicon Valley pioneers including Chris Anderson, editor of *Wired* magazine, and Evan Williams, founder of Blogger and Twitter, imposed strict limits on the use of technology for their own children. All of them had another thing in common: they required their children to read printed books. Alter analogizes the decision by these Silicon Valley pioneers to restrict their children's access to the very technology they invented to the motto of many successful drug dealers: "Don't get high on your own supply."

In a 2017 report for *60 Minutes,* reporter Anderson Cooper investigated the topic. He interviewed the few Silicon Valley executives who would admit their devices are designed to be addictive. These devices use complex algorithms to release dopamine in the brain. For example, most major social media platforms manipulate their programs and how they interact with users as a way of affecting the users' release of dopamine. In fact, companies now exist with the sole purpose of studying how to manipulate the reward center in the brain via your electronic device to maximize the release of dopamine. It's not practical, and many of us would be quite lonely if we were to live off the grid full-time. However, shutting your electronics off is an excellent spiritual tool. It is also incredibly empowering for you to manage your electronic devices rather than to let them manage you.

None of the spiritual tools presented here can work if your phone, iPad, or other electronic devices constantly distract you. So let's start with one of the most powerful spiritual tools you have possessed all along but have rarely used, *airplane mode.* By turning on airplane mode or otherwise shutting off your electronic devices for fifteen minutes or a half-hour during your morning ritual or at other times during the day, you give your brain a break and focus on *your* needs, not the needs of others. During this time you can journal, work out, meditate, or reflect—do whatever you want. Just make sure it is something that benefits your health and well-being. Over time, you may find the practice to be highly liberating and something you wish to incorporate more fully into your daily life.

When I first decided to try this I was terrified. The idea of shutting off my phone was not something I was comfortable with. However, I often thought about how, in my first attempt in the program, I received texts and calls all night long from friends who were still actively engaging in the lifestyle I walked away from years ago. These texts and calls kept me up at night and interfered with the quality of my sleep. They also triggered temptation in my mind, and I would sometimes linger in bed thinking about going out and meeting up with them and all the "fun" I would have.

With great trepidation, I put my phone in airplane mode at 9:00 p.m. and didn't turn it back on until after my morning meditation and workout. It was difficult at first but among the best things I ever did. It took a couple of weeks, but I began to sleep soundly and have less-stressful dreams. It became empowering to put my self-care and well-being over the needs of others. At this point, anyone who would call or text me between 11:00 p.m. and 5:00 a.m. without it being an emergency was not someone I wanted to know. My sleep improved, and so did my morning spiritual practice.

In the mornings, with my phone still off, I successfully established the habit of a full-body meditation and stretching in bed, coffee and a hot bath, reading *Just for Today* and *Daily Reflections,* eating a healthy breakfast, working out, and then turning off airplane mode. Without fail, as soon as I turn off airplane mode and get back on the grid, I get lots of texts, voicemails, and emails. I get inundated with the world and other people's issues and needs on a daily basis. On most days, the morning practice I have established as my daily norm puts me in a better mind-set to patiently deal with these issues. My morning practice sets the tone for the rest of my day and puts me in a state where I focus on gratitude. Usually, the positive energy stays with me for most of the day.

The Benefits of Meditation

Meditation is a critical spiritual tool because it helps control your monkey mind and, over time, helps reduce the tendency to act out in an impulsive way. Countless studies have confirmed that mindfulness meditation can improve emotional regulation,[219] reduce cravings for alcohol and other drugs, and greatly reduce stress and anxiety.[220] Even a half-hour or less a day has been proven to significantly reduce urges for alcohol, mind-altering drugs, and cigarettes.[221] These studies all reflect the long-term changes in brain function as a result of meditation. MRIs of the brain have confirmed that the amygdala—the primal region of our brain associated with our fight-or-flight instincts—appears to shrink when we meditate. As the amygdala shrinks, the prefrontal cortex, which is associated with higher brain function, including awareness, concentration, and decision making, thickens.[222] So, with all this evidence to support the positive role of meditation, it makes sense to integrate meditation into your nutritional, exercise, and twelve-step programs.

Mealtime Meditation

Many of us, myself included, gobble down our food as quickly as possible, given the demands of our day-to-day lives. When we were in active addiction, some of us went days at a time without eating, and when we did we often ate comfort foods to help ameliorate the hangover and tide us over until the next binge. As a result, whether we are in active addiction or in recovery, our relationship with food is dysfunctional. This includes not only what we are eating, but also how we eat it.

An effective way of staying present when you are eating your meal is to try a mealtime meditation. It takes time to get into the habit, but once the habit is established it almost becomes second nature. A mealtime meditation can be practiced when you are purchasing food, preparing food, and eating your meal. Follow this general framework:

- When **purchasing** food, turn on airplane mode and, if possible, try not to listen to music. Focus on where you are and think about what you are buying. Remember that what you are about to purchase will be going into your body and will have an effect on you. It will become part of you and will have either positive or negative consequences for you. Deciding which foods to buy is among the most important decisions you make every day.

- **Examine** the labels of the foods you like. If they contain high-fructose corn syrup or things you cannot pronounce, put them back and look for a healthier version. If you already set a nutritional goal, ask yourself whether what you are buying is consistent with that goal. Also ask yourself the following questions—not just once, but repeat them over and over, trying to coordinate the question with your breath. By repeating the question many times, it becomes a "mantra." A *mantra* is defined as a word or sound repeated to aid concentration in meditation.

- Is what I am buying something that will positively affect my blood work?
- Is it something that is consistent with my recovery principles?
- Is it something that is healthy for me?
- Is it something that is natural and comes from the earth?
- Is what I am about to buy consistent with my goals in recovery?
- With what I know about how sugar and caffeine affect my recovery, am I purchasing this product as a substitute?
- Was the product I am buying part of my "using diet"?
- Am I shopping emotionally?

■ While **preparing** your food, turn on airplane mode. Focus on what you are about to eat. What chemicals and compounds are contained in your food, and how do they impact your health? For the better? For the worse? Instead of thinking about where you are going later, whom you need to call, and what you did or did not do that day, really focus on what you are about to eat and focus on gratitude. Thank the farmer who grew your food, the people who cleaned it and harvested it, those who packaged it, the inspectors who ensured it is safe for you to eat, the truckers who transported it, and the people who made it available to you at the market. It takes a village to undertake all the necessary actions to put that meal on your table. Reflecting on that fact will reinforce just how interrelated we all are.

■ Give **thanks** for the food you are about to eat and focus on the nourishment the food will give your body. Thank yourself for taking the time to purchase and prepare healthy foods that will give you energy and enhance your physical appearance and mental focus, enabling you to live the life you want to live as a happy recovering person.

■ Here's a **sample meditation** that I have used when preparing my salad:

Thank you, God, for these fresh vegetables I am about to eat.
These vegetables give me the sustenance I need to get through my day.
These vegetables bring me energy and health and
promote wellness in my body and mind.
These vegetables are of this earth as I am of this earth.

I am grateful for this blessing and will remain
in gratitude throughout this day.

Use this meditation as an example or create your own. I happen to like corny meditations—you might, too.

- While **eating** meals, make sure to have airplane mode on to allow you to be present with your food. Your goal is to be conscious of each bite. Before eating, observe the colors of your food, smell the aroma, and check out the texture. While eating, chew slowly, focus on the taste and how it makes your mouth feel, focus on the changes as the food is masticated, and be grateful for the impulse to swallow, the process of swallowing, and how your body feels. After swallowing, just sit and notice how different your body feels. After your meal is done, do the same. Focus on how you felt at the beginning of your meal and after. What are your energy levels like? How have they changed? Do you feel good about what you ate? Was it easier to taste the food without distractions? If you are having a meal with loved ones, suggest that they participate in really putting thought into what they are eating as well.

This meditation is very potent for those who have quit smoking. A few weeks after I quit, I started to really taste my food again. Smoking harmed my ability to taste food, and as my taste buds healed when the toxins contained in cigarettes were removed, I realized I hadn't really tasted my food in a very long time.

Exercise Meditation

Your time at the gym is the perfect opportunity to provide both your body and mind with spiritual nourishment. Rather than having lots of distractions, it's best to put the phone on airplane mode, avoid calls and texts, and focus on yourself and your self-care. Whether weight training, taking a class, or doing cardio on your own, focus on your body. Focus on the specific muscles you are using and how they feel. Watch the muscles tighten and then relax. Focus on how that feels. Note the interrelationships among the various muscles in the body. For example, if you are working your biceps, notice how and when it contracts and what happens to your triceps. Notice what happens to your forearm. By focusing on the interrelationship of your muscles and how the body works, you'll have a greater appreciation for the miracle that is your body. Given that weight training involves repetitive movements, it's the perfect match for meditation.

Gym Meditation

It is easy to get distracted while working out, especially at the gym. Maybe we wind up cruising a hot guy or lady. Maybe we have issues at home or at the office. Everyone is under tremendous pressure these days—most of us are overwhelmed. When I get caught up on the mental baggage I carry around, I have a useful meditation to get me refocused on being present in the gym and not someplace else. You can give it a try and see if it works for you:

Stare into a mirror and look at yourself intensely. Confront yourself. Make sure you look yourself right in the eyes.

Ask yourself, "Why am I here at the gym?"

Ask yourself, "Am I focused on accomplishing my reason for being here?"

Ask yourself, "How deep do I want to take this workout?"

Keep asking yourself that question while looking yourself squarely in the eyes.

Tell yourself, "This is the only thing I am 100 percent in control of. This is all about the second part of the Serenity Prayer, "the courage to change the things I can." So how deep do I want to take this workout?"

By doing this meditation, you'll remind yourself that although in life you must often accept that which you cannot change, how you exercise and how intensely are completely in your control. There are few things in life to which the Serenity Prayer does not apply. How hard you exercise is one of them.

You can expand on these simple questions and turn this basic meditation into something much more.

Here's an example:

How deep do I want to take this workout?

When I was using, I had no energy, I felt like shit.

Exercise is liberating my body and soul!

I have energy again and I am excited to be alive.

So how deep do I want to take this?

Here's another example:
How deep do I want to take this?
I want to be able to dance at (my daughter's,
son's, cousin's, child's) wedding.
I am making my body and mind healthy for me,
my family, and all those who love me.
Exercise is liberating my body and soul!
So how deep do I want to take this?

And one more example:
How deep do I want to take this?
Addiction poisoned my body and mind.
The steps have taught me the way out.
Exercise is liberating my body and soul!
So how deep do I want to take this?

You can work in whatever goal you are trying to achieve. Notice the repetition of the core question and principle: "How deep do I want to take this?" and "Exercise is liberating my body and soul!" The meditation works as it helps keep the mind focused on goals and not the distractions that keep you from achieving them.

Full-Body Meditation

This can be practiced at any time of day. It works best in the morning. The meditation is extremely powerful, as it will help to remind you to stay in gratitude for all the things that make life so pleasurable, including having fingers, arms, shoulders, knees, hips, legs, and feet that work.

Remind yourself every morning: if you can scratch an itch on your own nose and wipe your own butt, you are incredibly blessed. If you see color, the landscape, and the faces of people you love, you are incredibly blessed. If you can walk to the store, church, work, or a twelve-step meeting, you are incredibly blessed. These are simple pleasures that many people don't feel gratitude for as a result of their years of active addiction and the damage they have done to their bodies and souls.

How blessed are you? It's gratitude for these simple pleasures that will help keep you sober. But you have to understand they are gifts that can be taken away by addiction or an unhealthy non-recovery-oriented lifestyle.

Remind yourself every morning: if you are waking up in your own bed, you are fortunate. You are among the lucky ones who are not incarcerated in a prison cell, a hospital, or a mental institution as a result of your active addiction. You get to wake up on soft sheets and a real mattress. How blessed are you? It's gratitude for these simple pleasures that will help keep you in recovery. But understand they are gifts that can be taken away by your addiction if you do not stay focused on your recovery.

Now let's get to the full-body meditation. Animals were my inspiration for this one. I have had three Persian cats in my life: Sable, Diva, and Gizmo. I also had one dog, a Chow-Akita mix named Los Angeles. All of them liked to sleep with me in bed. I noticed they all woke up in a similar way. They would wake up slowly, stretch all their paws, fully extend the front paws out and stretch their spines, then reverse and stretch in the other direction. They would wake slowly, deliberately, and stretch all their major muscle groups and then their energy center, the spine.

In active addiction, I would often wake up suddenly, not knowing what day it was; jump out of bed; curse like crazy; and rush to get going, totally stressed and anxious the whole time. I would chain-smoke cigarettes, and if I had a little coke lying around, I would use that for a brief yet unsustainable burst of energy. Now, I take my time getting out of bed and do a full-body meditation from my head down every morning. It's a great way to start the day. Here's how it goes:

- Start with your head. Give thanks for your brain, eyes, nose, and mouth. When focusing on a specific body part, for example, the eyes, open and close them and feel the movement. Reflect on how your life would be different without a properly functioning set of eyes. How about your nose? Imagine if you had no sense of smell. Your mouth? Think about not being able to taste your food.
- Work your way down your arms, fingers, lungs, heart, stomach, genitals, legs, feet, and toes. As you are making your way down, meditate on specific body parts. Stretch that body part. Take a deep breath with your lungs. Really deep breathe; get all the stale air out. Inhale as much fresh air as you can. Put your hand on your chest and

feel your lungs and chest expand and contract. Reflect on the miracle of your own heart beating. I often think about how much cocaine I used to do. I am grateful my heart did not explode. I am also grateful that the chest pains I had for the six months of recovery went away. I am grateful my heart is healthy and I take care of it. Reflect back on your history of using and modify as appropriate for you.

- Stretch your energy center, your spine, as much as possible—backward, forward, like a cat or dog. Sense how your body feels different after you stretch your spine.

You can come up with your own variations of this morning meditation. It's subjective, so do whatever works for you. The thing to keep in mind is that everything else is really irrelevant without a healthy body. Ask a billionaire with terminal cancer if she would give all her money up to have her health back—I bet she would. This meditation will remind you every morning of how wealthy you are as you wake up in a body that works.

Some people may want to take things a little deeper. If this is you, here are some examples for the heart, fingers, and eyes:

Heart: Place your hand over your chest and gently feel your heart beating.
Thank you to my heart,
Which works even while my mind sleeps,
Which sends oxygen and life to the rest of my body,
Which has continued to love and nourish me even when I did not love and nourish it,
Which I cannot live without.
I will remain mindful today of how my heart enables my body to function and maintain life. I will remember to nurture my heart and remain grateful.

Fingers: Stretch your fingers gently as you say this meditation:
My fingers make so much possible,
They work together so miraculously,
They benefit me at work and at play,

They are beautiful creations without which my life would be much more difficult.

I will remain mindful today of how frequently I use my fingers. I will remember to nurture them, and I will remain grateful.

Eyes: Close your eyes to begin, and open your eyes during the meditation.

Without my eyes, my world is dark, and I live in shadows.

With my eyes, I see the world in vibrant colors and enjoy the splendor of my higher power's creation.

I want to enjoy the full color of living for the rest of my life.

I will remain mindful today of how much pleasure my eyes bring. I will remember to nurture them, and I will remain grateful.

Active Fellowship at Your Home Group

By becoming a fellowship coordinator or "social chair" at your home group, you can set up fun, active activities for everyone to participate in. If your home group does not have a social chair, you can petition the group to create the position and volunteer to fill it. You can become the change you want to see in yourself and others by taking the lead in integrating the principles of Spiritual Adrenaline into "active fellowship." For example, how about having fellowship at a farmer's market or going out for hikes or to the beach? The different types of active fellowship are endless, and I bet others will be open-minded and willing to participate.

Meeting Meditation

I often see people at meetings relentlessly texting, gobbling down cookies with coffee, or looking anxious and stressed about having to actually sit still for an hour or for seventy-five or ninety minutes. I can relate to this because it describes me for a very long time in early recovery. I started the bad habit of zoning out when "How It Works" was read at the beginning of a meeting, and I would think about everything else but what was being read and where I was. I developed meeting meditations to alleviate anxiety and stress caused by having to sit still in a room filled with strangers, which helped me to share honestly from deep inside me. These meditations are also designed to refocus the mind back to gratitude.

"How It Works" Meditation

If you tend to lose focus when "How It Works" is read at a meeting, take a deep breath, inhale, exhale, and, with each breath, ask yourself these questions:

- *"Why am I here?"* Continue breathing and ponder the answer to that question. On the inhale, ask the question; on the exhale, answer it. Among the answers may be "because I love myself," "I love my family," or "I deserve to be happy."

- *"My life is better in sobriety because . . ."* Continue to breathe deeply and reflect on all the gifts of your sobriety: maybe because you have a job, your family, or your health, or because you are in recovery just for today. Be grateful for a life without hangovers, your bills being paid, your health getting better, your loved ones learning to respect you, and the opportunity to be of service to others who are sick and suffering.

- *"I dedicate this meeting to . . ."* Continue to breathe deeply, and if you don't want to be at the meeting, dedicate the meeting or your presence at the meeting to a family member, spouse, child, partner, or anyone else who benefits from your recovery. Keep repeating, "I dedicate this meeting to . . ." over and over while "How It Works" is being read.

The remaining meeting meditations permit you to meditate on behalf of others. This is a form of service that benefits both you and the other person.

- *"I see in you a spiritual awakening and thank you for being here to share your recovering spirit."* Continue to breathe deeply in and out and look at each person in the room. One person at a time while breathing in and out, repeat that phrase. Keep in mind the mere fact that these individuals who have taken the first step and attend meetings all have had a spiritual awakening, whether they realize it or not.

- *"You are the promises of the program in living form, and for your gift I am grateful."* When people put their hand up to announce their day count or anniversary, take a deep breath in and out for that person and repeat: "You are the promises of the program in living form, and for your gift I am grateful." See in the gift of counting days or the celebration of an anniversary that person's spiritual awakening and the fact that the promises of the Twelve Steps do come true if we work the program. This simple meeting meditation will keep you in gratitude.

- *"Breathe in the suffering of others and breathe out loving kindness."* A final type of meeting meditation is to listen to the shares of others who are sick and suffering. When they share about their anxiety, fear, resentment, cravings, or character defects, take a deep breath in and take in their suffering. You are in a way sucking the suffering away from them. Next, exhale deeply and with the exhale send them empathy, loving kindness, gratitude, and love. Continue to breathe in and out and practice this meditation until the person finishes sharing.

Supreme Teacher

The Buddhist concept of supreme teacher is a most useful tool and can turn what you perceive as an unpleasant and/or unwelcome experience into one from which you learn and grow. This concept can be applied to people, places, or things that are out of your control and are perceived to be oppressing you. Rather than just accepting what you cannot change, the supreme teacher concept asks you to go a step further. It asks that you express gratitude for the lack of control, even if you perceive the person, place, or things as negative. Why be grateful for an asshole who is abusing you or someone who is being unfair to you? By seeing this behavior as a teachable moment, a way you can learn and grow, you learn to find gratitude in what used to make you feel oppressed, act out, and later feel guilty about it. This change in your mind-set and view of the situation can teach you humility, compassion, patience, and other virtues in ways you never before thought possible. When you learn to convert a perceived oppressor into a supreme teacher, you recognize that your perceived suffering can be turned into gratitude. This helps you keep loving kindness in your heart even for your actual or perceived worst oppressors. You can avoid anger and resentment, which triggers and feeds your addiction and your suffering.

The Dalai Lama often refers to the Chinese as his supreme teachers. Decades ago, China invaded Tibet, brutally oppressed the Tibetan Buddhist community, and attempted to erase thousands of years of Buddhist history. China installed its own Dalai Lama who presides from Beijing, and China forced the Tibetan Dalai Lama (the one recognized all around the world except by China and North Korea) into exile in India. Even after all of this, the Dalai Lama prays for the Chinese and keeps loving kindness and compassion for them in his heart.

The Dalai Lama is grateful to the Chinese for reminding him that even though he is the Dalai Lama, he is still of human flesh and not in control of all the actions and consequences in the world. The Dalai Lama says the Chinese teach him humility, patience, and empathy. He practices forgiveness toward them to avoid anger, which would serve no purpose other than to destroy him and, by association, his followers and their ancient and timeless spiritual tradition.

If we are able to practice this tool in our daily affairs, it helps take us beyond white-knuckle acceptance, anger, and lingering resentments. It helps us learn from uncomfortable or painful situations and permits us to practice loving kindness unimpeded by life on life's terms.

The principle works with small stuff, too—lesser things that can lead to really major resentments. For example, I practice this principle almost every day as I walk around Hell's Kitchen in New York City. My neighborhood is adjacent to Times Square and crowded with tourists almost all of the time. They block sidewalks, stop right in front of me to take pictures, and travel in herds, making it almost impossible to navigate quickly around them, especially during the holidays. I used to curse these folks and wish that unpleasant things would happen to them. Now I laugh, look up at the sky, and thank my higher power for reminding me that the universe does not revolve around me. It reminds me that I am only one of billions of other living beings on this planet and I must learn to share. I also think about how blessed I am to live in a place where people from all over the world come to gaze in wonder at its beauty.

Naps

Your body is not designed to get up in the morning and go all day without a break. It naturally wants to rest for a brief period halfway through the

day in order to awaken energized and refreshed. A quick nap can work
wonders to pull you through a sleep-deprived day. A 2008 study found
that a forty-five-minute daytime nap improves memory and overall body
function. Other studies have found that naps can lower blood pressure.
Researchers at Harvard Medical School have come up with advice on how
to take a "good nap."[223] Here are their recommendations:

- Keep it short. The twenty- to thirty-minute nap may be the ideal
  pick-me-up. Napping for even just a few minutes has benefits.
  Longer naps can lead to sleep inertia—the postsleep grogginess that
  can be difficult to shake off.

- Find a dark, quiet, cool place. You don't want to waste a lot of time
  getting to sleep. Reducing light and noise helps most people nod off
  faster. Cool temperatures are helpful, too.

- Plan on it. Waiting until daytime sleepiness gets so bad that you
  have to take a nap can be uncomfortable and dangerous if, say,
  you're driving. A regular nap time may also help you get to sleep
  faster and wake up quicker.

- Time your caffeine. Caffeine takes some time to kick in. A Japanese
  study published several years ago found that drinking a caffeinated
  beverage and then taking a short nap immediately afterward was the
  most restful combination because the sleep occurred just before the
  caffeine took effect. I'm not so sure about that approach—the mere
  suggestion of caffeine, in the form of coffee taste or smell, wakes me
  up. Regardless of the exact timing, you need to coordinate caffeine
  intake with your nap.

- Don't feel guilty! The well-timed nap can make you more productive
  at work and at home.

Napping can be a game changer. Rather than ingesting unsustainable
energy sources from caffeine, starch, and sugar, taking a twenty-minute nap
can give you the needed recharge naturally. Rather than continuing to push
your body beyond its capabilities, learn to respect its limits and rest when
you need to. Sleep deprivation makes it easier to grab for junk food, booze,
or drugs, and that, of course, can contribute to weight gain.[224] *New York
Times* reporter Anahad O'Connor reported on various studies that linked

lack of sleep with weight gain.[225] These studies found that sleep deprivation can cause weight gain because it triggers people to eat more. In his study, Matthew P. Walker, PhD, University of California, Berkeley, wrote:

> A sleepy brain appears to not only respond more strongly to junk food, but also has less ability to rein that impulse in. . . . The underlying effects of sleep deprivation on the body can in many ways be pronounced. The stress hormone cortisol climbs, and markers of inflammation rise. Hormones that stimulate appetite increase, while hormones that blunt it drop.[226]

Dr. Walker found that without enough rest, adenosine builds up and may start to degrade communication between networks in the brain. Dr. Walker described sleeping as the equivalent of rebooting the brain. Dr. Walker's findings are another example of how our physical and psychological health are mutually dependent.

Music

Music is a powerful spiritual tool that can play a positive or negative role in your recovery. There has been extensive research on the complex relationship between addiction and music. In 2012, researchers studying the impact of music on the brain function of people in recovery published their report in *The Journal of Music Therapy and Addictions*. The researchers found that music "holds many important emotional and social functions. It is intertwined with the issues we must deal with."[227] Those with substance use disorders often tend to "be drawn with great yearning, back to their drug-abuse-related music."[228]

You can take music with you anywhere. You can integrate music into your recovery in a positive manner that enhances your recovery by reinforcing positive messages of health, hope, and healing.

The Soundtrack of Your Life

Inventory your "using playlist." This is the music you listened to when drinking or using drugs with friends. Sit down and write out the artists, songs, and messages. Think about how frequently you listened to that music when you were using and about how the messages contained in the music affected you emotionally. Reflect on whether or not the music encouraged you to use and what other negative behaviors were associated with your using soundtrack. Ask yourself these questions:

- Does the music define my personal, social, and ethnic identity?
- How do I use music in my daily life?
- How does music relate to my past substance abuse?
- Does my music contain negative messaging that reinforces depression or isolation?
- Does my music glorify substance use and/or abuse?

Commit to putting this music and these songs and artists on hold until you can get a solid foundation for your recovery.

Next, reflect back on your childhood, your formative years, or some other point in your life when you were happy. Think about the music you listened to then that made you happy—the soundtrack of your life before you started abusing mind-altering substances. What music and songs made you happy? What songs rekindle positive memories in your life? Inventory this music and these songs and develop a soundtrack for your recovery—music and songs that bring back favorable memories, suggest positive aspirations, and lift you up.

When I was in active addiction, I almost never listened to new music. I was stuck in the same people, places, and things, and that included music.

In recovery, it's important to grow and expand your existing comfort zones. Download Pandora or some other music service and listen to various stations. Develop an entirely new soundtrack of music and songs consistent with your goals in sobriety. I listen to Pandora all the time and I am constantly downloading new music. Listening to new music that is upbeat puts me in a positive mood. Rather than being stale, the music I listen to is fresh and constantly changing.

Dancing

I am a terrible dancer and rarely dance in public. I often sing and dance in my apartment or in the gym if no one else is around. When I am at weddings and other events, people often try to pull me out onto the dance floor. I try as hard as possible to avoid getting pulled out. The sad thing about this is that I actually want to do it. I am just nervous as hell and focused on other people judging me. I am sure no one else cares, and likely most would never even notice. I do know that when I dance, I feel liberated and so much better. A number of people I know in recovery go to sunrise "pop-up" dances and swear by them. There is something incredibly liberating about letting it all go and dancing.

In an article available on soberrecovery.com, one person described dancing this way: "Dance, being the most fundamental and unique form of art, affects people spiritually first. Then it refines them socially and physically. As a form of therapy it not only helps people with chronic illnesses, it also helps socially and physically abused people to cope with their emotions, anger, and frustration on a mental level."[229]

Recent studies have confirmed that dancing can play a useful role in the treatment and rehabilitation of people in recovery. These studies have concluded that dancing works by raising self-esteem through an improved relationship with your body. Over time, this comfort with one's own body translates to greater confidence overall and an ability to combat addiction.[230]

So my recommendation is to dance in the shower, at home, at the gym, on the way to meetings, and any other time you want to. Some might call this dancing through life.

Gratitude Trips

Can you remember taking vacations in active addiction? Did you come to the realization either then or after you got into recovery that it did not really matter where you went, because the bottles and bars looked basically the same wherever you were? If you were in a bar in Hawaii it might have been warmer and have a prettier view, but once you were loaded you could be in downtown Flint, Michigan, because the bottom of a bottle looked the same and you probably wouldn't remember it anyway.

In a self-care-based recovery, I suggest that you vacation and travel in an entirely different way. Your vacations should be in places filled with activities that are consistent with your new lifestyle and healthy and spiritually fulfilling self-care goals.

I call these vacations "gratitude trips." They are intended to be a reward for your new way of living and they reinforce, rather than undercut, your recovery. Here are a few examples:

- **Spiritual Adrenaline Adventures:** If you visit my website, you'll see that I lead active adventures that combine nutrition, exercise, and spirituality. For example, there is a five-day hike on the Incan Trail to Machu Picchu, hiking in the Grand Canyon, glacier climbing in Banff National Park in the Canadian Rockies and, soon, a trek to Salzburg, Austria, for a *Sound of Music*–themed adventure and hike in the Austrian Alps.

- **Yoga of Twelve-Step Recovery Retreats (Y12SR):** Y12SR is a brilliant program founded by Nikki Myers. Any of her retreats are highly recommended. Her annual retreat in the Blue Hills of North Carolina is truly wonderful. At Y12SR retreats, you will meet other local leaders in the movement to integrate yoga with the Twelve Steps of addiction recovery.

- **IntenSati:** Patricia Moreno organizes frequent intensive retreats that focus on physical fitness and bringing out the leader inside you. Any of her retreats will change the way you look at your life and your world.

- **Recovery 2.0:** Tommy Rosen's online community, Recovery 2.0, also offers retreats both in the United States and abroad. It's an excellent place to meet other like-minded people who understand that recovery is based upon a strong foundation in self-care.

- **Yoga of Recovery:** Yoga of Recovery holds affordable weekend and weeklong workshops that focus on integrating yoga and Ayurveda into a twelve-step practice.

- **Roundups:** A number of twelve-step groups sponsor local events called roundups. These events bring together like-minded people to enjoy meetings and topical workshops, often including meditation, fellowship, nutrition, and exercise. They are really fun.

You don't have to go on an organized adventure or retreat or spend a lot of money on your gratitude trips. There are weekend retreats that are economical at KTD Monastery in Woodstock, New York, or other Buddhist monasteries around the country. Another affordable weekend retreat, if you can get to New England, is at the birthplace of Bill Wilson in East Dorset, Vermont. You can attend a meeting in the building where Bill was born, have communal meals, stay over at the Wilson House B&B, and visit the graves of Bill and Lois Wilson.

All over the country and the world, you can find similar places to meditate and contemplate. Any natural preserve or park where you can connect to nature serves a similar purpose. Check out Arches or Bryce Canyon National Park in the U.S., and your concept of the universe and our place in it will never be the same.

If you think you cannot afford to treat yourself, think again. Just the way you found the money in active addiction to destroy your life, you can put your money in sobriety toward things that can improve your life. For example, the money I used to purchase cigarettes is put into a gratitude vacation fund. I estimate the cost of cigarettes when I was smoking at $20.00 per day. I smoked a pack and a half a day and they cost about $15.00 a pack when I quit in New York City. My cigarette habit added up to about $7,300.00 a year.

I put that money toward trips that permit me to celebrate my emancipation from the mental slavery of smoking, cocaine, alcohol, Xanax, and other substances. Some of the trips funded by the money I used to give to Philip Morris to slowly poison me are vacations, including Machu Picchu in Peru; a surfing-yoga retreat in Costa Rica; hiking 21,000 feet to the summit of Mount Kilimanjaro; climbing Mount Rainier; hiking to the base camp of Mount Everest; visiting the birthplace of Buddha in Nepal; visiting the exact location where Buddha found enlightenment under the Bodhi Tree in India. All of these are adventures that challenged my lungs. I would not have been capable of doing any of these excursions had I continued to smoke. While traveling I journal, review my journals from the past, and work on gratitude lists. There is nothing more spiritual for me than being an ex-smoker, climbing some of the tallest mountains in the world, and taking a deep breath from my healthy lungs as I enjoy the view.

Reading

Reading spiritual literature is a powerful tool that can profoundly change your outlook on life and your recovery. Reading something that relates to you and can benefit you in your life is a reminder of the interrelated nature of the common human experience. In *Coming Out Spiritually,* author Christian de la Huerta describes reading as "an effective technique for escaping the confinement of our minds."[231]

De la Huerta recommends early-morning reading. He says, "I frequently start out the day by reading something inspirational that will anchor my consciousness in a positive context and remind me of a larger or global view. This inevitably has the effect of bringing my concerns into perspective; it reminds me that I am not alone, that there are others out there who share a sense of mission, urgency, and understanding about what is going on here on our plane at this time."

Spiritual Adrenaline Inspiration: Kyczy H., California

Kyczy H. has long-term recovery and is the author of *Life in Bite-Sized Morsels, Yoga and the Twelve-Step Path,* and *Yogic Tools for Recovery: A Guide to Working the Twelve Steps.* In addition to her books and managing a yoga studio, she actively participates in Yoga of Twelve Step Recovery, or Y12SR. Here's what she said about how yoga has helped her and can help you:

> The practice and study of yoga brought me back from the precipice of relapse. The Twelve Steps got me into my second decade of recovery, but deeper issues, not cognitive in nature, needed to be addressed. Yoga helped me discover those. In moving my story out of my head in through my body I have healed harms that I had long forgotten.
>
> Yoga practice and philosophy have deepened my reverence for utilizing the Twelve Steps as a method for uncovering issues that disturb me and my relationships. Using yoga philosophy and models gives me a new insight into ways to address the human condition. Active addiction turned up the volume on these problems; yoga can help turn it down. The philosophy gave me a framework for doing the steps, and breathing, asanas, and meditation helped to unify the wellness as it grew.
>
> Anxiety, stress, and fear are all kinds of "out of body" experiences. They are out of real time (past or future) and can swirl away any composure one has in dealing with the present

moment. Breath is the key to reinhabiting the body. Yoga philosophy can help heal the mind; the breath moves this new awareness to the nervous system and the body. Addiction separated me from that connection between my feelings and my mind. Awareness of my breathing can unify me and my senses. Control of my breath permits better control of the mind. It allows me to be quiet and make better choices in my life. Breathe slowly, with kindness, and heal.

Here's a list of the spiritual tools I have discussed in this chapter:

- Airplane mode
- Mealtime meditations
- Exercise meditations
- Full-body meditation
- Active fellowship
- Meeting meditations
- Supreme teacher
- Naps
- Music: the soundtrack of your life
- Gratitude trips
- Reading spiritual literature

CHAPTER TWELVE

The Seven-Day Spiritual Adrenaline Detox

Congratulations. If you've gotten this far you've invested substantial time in reading this book and set yourself up for success by following my recommendations relating to starting your day-one baseline. Seize the day! A new life begins outside your comfort zone. If you don't know how to get there, the tools of Spiritual Adrenaline and the seven-day detox practiced with the Twelve Steps will provide a strong foundation for success.

This seven-day detox works for anyone—whether you are new to recovery or you simply want to jump-start your program.

Nutrition

It's time to make your nutritional habits a thing of the past and surrender to the fact that you can't eat whatever unhealthy foods you want whenever you want. That's the first step!

The Nutritional Solution: Addiction Paleo with More Complex Carbs

I recommend a diet that is relatively high in protein and fat, with more complex carbohydrates than standard Paleo approaches. This is because I'm taking into account your years of active addiction, the likelihood you came into recovery malnourished, and because transitioning suddenly to the 10 percent or less of total calories from carbohydrates that ketogenic diets recommend is unhealthy for newcomers.

Rather than focusing on a percentage of your daily calories that come from carbs, as I've noted, I recommend you eat carbohydrates in *moderation* for breakfast, your morning snack, and/or lunch. I also recommend you cut the carbs off in midafternoon, about 3:00 to 5:00 p.m., and eat only proteins and healthy fats after that. Here's why.

Protein is the building block of your body and represents 10 to 20 percent of body mass, depending on your age, weight, and overall health. Protein increases your metabolic rate and helps to reduce appetite while providing a consistent source of energy without spiking blood sugar.[232]

Fats have been unfairly maligned by the processed foods industry that has been relentlessly marketing "low-fat," high-sugar foods. Fats in your diet are actually necessary for your body to function properly.[233] Fats play a critical role in digestion by serving as the essential element for the transportation and absorption of vitamins A, D, E, and K.[234] Fat cells also serve as insulation to maintain proper body temperature and as a source of energy in times of caloric need after depletion of sugar and carbohydrates. Most importantly, for those in detox, healthy fats help reduce cravings and stabilize your blood sugar while providing energy.

A 2011 Princeton University study found that the severity of withdrawal in alcoholics and addicts had a direct correlation with the nutrients in their diet in active addiction and while going through withdrawal.[235] Research has shown that a diet high in fat will help avoid spikes in your blood sugar,[236] while providing the nourishment your organs and body need.

Recommended sources of lean protein include chicken; sirloin steak; 90 percent grass-fed beef; pork; turkey; and fish. By choosing lean protein sources, those in the detox process can often eat a healthier version of their favorite comfort foods. Turkey burgers, lean hamburgers, and chicken sandwiches are healthful and delicious substitutes for your favorite comfort foods. Now in a healthier form, these foods can go from part of the problem to part of the solution.

Organ Health

If you have liver disease or issues with any other organs, you may want to avoid red meats to reduce stress and inflammation on your organs while you detox. Substantial protein intake can take a toll on already-stressed organs. Talk with your doctor about having blood work done to ascertain the health of your liver, kidneys, pancreas, lungs, and heart prior to integrating the nutritional recommendations in this or any other guide.

- **Fats:** Recommended sources of these fats include oily fish such as salmon, mackerel, sardines, trout, and herring. Nuts, seeds, and beans that are high in omega oils include poppy, grape, sunflower, hemp, corn, wheat germ, cottonseed, and soybeans. You can get healthy fats not only from the foods you eat, but also during the preparation process. Cook with extra virgin olive oil or coconut oil, and you just improved your diet. Olive oil and fresh lemon juice also make a great salad dressing, and olive oil and a little balsamic vinegar make a delicious dip. These modest adjustments can have a major positive impact on your health over time.

- **Carbs:** People in recovery should consume complex carbs every day. My recommendation is to cut off carbs between 3:00 and 5:00 p.m., as mentioned earlier. If that is too early, set your own cutoff at 7:00 p.m. or 8:00 p.m. and then slowly try to move it earlier. If you are counting calories, I recommend daily intake from complex carbs in the range of 20 to 30 percent of your total calories. I strongly recommend that if you are in detox or in early recovery, you stay away from processed and starchy carbs and favor complex carbs. How do you know a complex carb? It's simple: if nature created it, it's likely a complex carb. If it's man-made, it's probably not. Plenty of complex carbs can become healthy comfort foods. Sweet potato can become sweet potato fries, pie, or pancakes. There are many recipes available online to help you create new and healthy forms of your favorite comfort foods. Check out www.delish.com, www.allrecipes.com, www.eatingwell.com, and www.expnutrition.com.

- **Coffee and Caffeine:** Keep your coffee intake limited to one or two cups a day. Try to get used to coffee without sugar. Rather, sweeten with one of my recommended substitutes, some of which are even sweeter than sugar. Caffeine can contribute to a cycle of ups and downs, especially when combined with lots of sugar.

Vitamins and Minerals

Check with your doctor about taking a quality multivitamin daily (with no added preservatives, sugar, or artificial colors). Although all vitamins are important to the proper functioning of your body, for the purposes of this guide I recommend you focus on vitamins A, B, C, and D. If you eat our recommended *detox superfoods,* you will have the peace of mind that you are providing your body with almost all the vitamins and minerals it needs naturally.

Detox Superfoods

You don't need to concern yourself with eating all organic or vegan. If you choose to, more power to you. *The important thing is that you eat three to four healthy meals a day with healthy snacks in between.* If you don't care for kale, for example, eat asparagus. If you don't like chicken, substitute turkey or salmon.

I have broken down the detox superfoods into each of the groups in the chart below. Since it is specifically intended for people doing the seven-day detox, this list is more limited than the superfoods list I provided in an earlier chapter. I've also included foods that will provide your body with the vitamins and minerals necessary to stimulate hormone production. Here you go!

Food	What It Has[1]	How It Helps
Group 1: Antioxidants		
Apple	Vitamin C, **dietary fiber**, khellin, flavonoids, polyphenols, pantothenic acid	Antioxidants, energy, blood sugar stabilization
Orange	Vitamins B and C, **fiber**, folate, copper, calcium, pantothenic acid, magnesium	Antioxidants, energy, blood-sugar stabilization

1 This list is not intended to be all-inclusive. Rather, my intent is to provide a snapshot of the spectrum of nutrients you will receive if you incorporate one food from each group daily. Given the high mineral content in some of these foods, it is highly recommended that those with liver or kidney issues have their blood tested to ascertain organ health.

Food	What It Has	How It Helps
Blueberry	Vitamins A, C, K; calcium, flavonoids, potassium, polyphenols, pantothenic acid, magnesium, zinc	Antioxidants, energy, blood-sugar stabilization
Group 2: Healthy Fat		
Pumpkin Seeds	Beta-carotene, beta-cryptoxanthin, tyrosine, tryptophan, lutein, linoleic acid, vitamin E	Prompts hormone production, restores muscle; nutrients for organ function, energy
Flaxseed	Omega-3, magnesium, tryptophan, thiamine, linoleic acid, vitamin E	Energy, hormone production, mood
Avocado	Glutamine, vitamin B6, folic acid, vitamin E, pantothenic acid, glutathione	Energy, hormone production, mood
Almonds	Tyrosine, omega-3	Energy, hormone production, mood
Olive Oil	Oleic acid, fatty acid, polyphenols	Energy, antioxidants, mood, hormone production, blood-sugar stabilization
Group 3: Leafy Greens		
Spinach	Free-form amino acids, l-glutamine, folic acid	Energy, restores muscle, proper organ function, mood, hormone production, blood-sugar stabilization
Kale/Asparagus	Folic acid, thiamine, calcium, vitamins E and K	Energy, mood, hormone production, blood-sugar stabilization
Group 4: Proteins		
Fish/Chicken/Turkey[2]	Tryptophan and 5-HTP, thiamine, tyrosine, folic acid, niacin, branched-chain amino acids, choline, pantothenic acid, creatine	Energy, mood, hormone production, blood-sugar stabilization

2 Vegans or vegetarians can substitute plant-based protein (which is expensive) or substitute beans for these meats as a protein source. A word of caution: if you are substituting beans, watch the carbohydrate intake so your total nutrient intake is kept in balance.

Food	What It Has	How It Helps
Group 5: Complex Carbs		
Sweet Potato	Beta-carotene, vitamin A, omega-3, omega-6, magnesium, vitamins C and B6, potassium, **dietary fiber,** niacin	Energy, brain and organ function, mood, assists muscle growth and maintenance, blood-sugar stabilization, hormone production
Brown Rice	Vitamins B1, B3, B6; magnesium, thiamine, niacin, iron, phosphorus, **dietary fiber,** selenium, copper	Energy, brain and organ function, mood, assists muscle growth and maintenance, blood-sugar stabilization, hormone production
Water		
Water (minimum two gallons each day)	None, but necessary to break down and carry nutrients to cells and for almost all functions at the cellular level (mineral water contains some nutrients, but not addressed here)	Necessary for all body functions: energy, mood, hormone production, etc.

All of the foods suggested above are available at supermarkets and most are relatively inexpensive. I recommend that you eat at least one item from each of Groups 1 through 5 every day as part of your detox regimen. I also recommend incorporating my recovery superspices in your morning, afternoon, and late-night snacks. When you eat three or four meals a day along with healthy snacks, it should not be challenging to eat from the first five groups. You can integrate these healthy food choices into your existing diet and phase out the less healthy choices over time. If you do this, you can have the peace of mind that you are providing your body with the nutritional self-care it needs.

In this book, I do not provide portion size. My only advice is something those in addiction recovery do not like to hear: moderation. Megadoses of any vitamin, mineral, supplement, food, or other substance will hurt rather than help. Megadoses put your organs under stress and cause inflammation. Since you likely stressed your organs while using, you don't want to continue to do that in recovery. Use moderation and check the recommended daily allowance for each food group. You can find the recommended allowances at www.health.gov/dietaryguidelines.

Water

I recommend two gallons of water for an adult every day in detox. That's a lot of water, I know; but you are detoxing! Water is a critical component of every single body function and the conduit by which you help remove toxins and restore balance to your body.[237]

In his book *Water: You're Not Sick, You're Thirsty,* Fereydoon Batmanghelidj, MD, explains why a lack of water in our bodies can affect our emotional state and trigger depression. Dr. Batmanghelidj says that at times of emotional stress, the brain goes into overdrive in an attempt to deal with the overload of emotion. As part of the brain's reaction, it requires substantial amounts of water to act as a conduit for the transfer of energy to fuel brain function. Dr. Batmanghelidj writes that the "depressive state caused by dehydration can lead to chronic fatigue syndrome."[238] My recommendation is to drink pure water often, and as much as you can.

Smoking

If you are trying to quit smoking, I recommend reading *Allen Carr's Easy Way to Stop Smoking* during this seven-day detox. You can smoke while you read it, so what do you have to lose? Carr's book has sold more than thirteen million copies and it has helped many people quit.

Avoid Too Much Sugar

Avoid overeating Group 1 foods, as they are high in fructose. Even though sugar naturally occurs in fruit, eating excessive amounts will cause your blood sugar to spike and then drop, and increase mood swings and cravings—exactly what you want to avoid.

Additionally, remember that juicing is also not recommended, as it removes fiber from fruits and vegetables. Without the fiber, your body will not be able to absorb the nutrients as effectively. Moreover, without chewing and the process of breaking down the nutrients in your mouth, juicing can provide a massive sugar rush in seconds, without your body absorbing nutrients. That's why I recommend eating the fruit or vegetable rather than juicing. If you are going to juice, I recommend juicing green veggies rather than fruit.

If you are buying fruit or vegetable juice, be wary of those containing added sugar. Studies have linked the extremely high sugar content in fruit juices to obesity and diabetes.[239] If you buy fruit juice at the market, mix it with water. A good rule of thumb is one-quarter cup of juice to every cup of water. You can add stevia to give the juice-water mixture more sweetness and flavor.

Morning Cleanse

Incorporate my recovery superfoods into your current diet rather than replacing your diet outright with my recommendations. In the morning, put the recovery superspices to work along with low-glycemic-load sugar substitutes to cleanse your body over the course of the day. I recommend that you do this morning cleanse every day as part of a commitment to establish a morning spiritual practice. While drinking your cleanse, why not write in your spiritual journal or read *Just for Today, Daily Reflections,* or other recovery-related literature that you enjoy and benefit from?

I recommend rotating every morning between the two morning-cleanse cocktails. On Sunday, you can drink your favorite or experiment with suggested recovery superspices to create your own.

Monday, Wednesday, Friday
1 cup almond milk (unsweetened)
2 tablespoons cinnamon or nutmeg
1 tablespoon minced garlic or garlic powder
Honey, agave, or stevia to taste

Preparation: Heat one cup of almond milk slowly. As it is heating, stir in one tablespoon each of cinnamon or nutmeg. Add in garlic powder and stir. Add any of the recover

Tuesday, Thursday, Saturday
2 teaspoons cumin powder
2 teaspoons fennel seeds
1 lemon, cut in half
1 cup water

Preparation: Boil water, and when boiling add the cumin and fennel. Stir well and then turn heat off and let sit until it cools. Stir occasionally. Squeeze juice of one fresh lemon into the mixture and stir well. Strain to remove seeds, and drink. Add any of the recovery sweetener substitutes—honey, agave, or stevia—to taste, but a maximum of one teaspoon at this point. Any sweetener should be limited to about a teaspoon or a teaspoon and a half given the number of carbs and calories.

I recommend making five cups of these cleanses at a time and storing your cleanses in the refrigerator to save time.

Midday Cleanse

With your lunch or any time during the middle of the day, provide your body with a powerful antioxidant cleanse with matcha tea. Mix your matcha with your choice of nutmeg, nonalcoholic vanilla, or cinnamon, and add in one of your optional recovery sweeteners to taste. Trader Joe's sells a tasty vanilla flavoring that is alcohol free. I also recommend Frontier Natural Products' nonalcoholic vanilla flavoring. It's absolutely delicious and will provide your body with a natural potent healer that will enhance your detox and your efforts to establish conscious contact with your body.

If you are not a fan of matcha, substitute green or chamomile tea but add in my recovery superspices and sweeteners.

Evening Cleanse

Your evening cleanse becomes part of the commitment to establishing an evening spiritual practice. While drinking your cleanse, write in your spiritual journal about the day, complete your Tenth Step inventory, and if you can, also prepare a gratitude list. You can read *Just for Today, Daily Reflections,* or any other recovery-related literature that you enjoy.

I recommend rotating every evening between the two recommended cleanse cocktails. On Sunday, you can drink your favorite or experiment with recovery superspices to create your own. The evening cleanse is intended to help your body eliminate toxins as you sleep, repair itself, and get ready for the day ahead while stimulating your metabolism to enhance weight loss.

Monday, Wednesday, Friday

1 teaspoon turmeric
1 teaspoon garlic

1 cup soy, coconut, or almond milk

Stevia, agave, or other recovery supersweetener, to a maximum of 1½ teaspoon

Preparation: Heat soy, coconut, or almond milk slowly. Once heated, stir in turmeric and garlic. Stir well while heating. Remove from heat, let cool, and stir in your optional recovery supersweetener, being mindful of the quantity—maximum of 1½ teaspoon.

For this cleanse, I do not recommend preparing multiple cleanses ahead of time. This cleanse tastes and stays better if prepared and immediately consumed.

Tuesday, Thursday, Saturday

Ginger root (½ cup shredded root)

½ lemon (squeeze juice into mix and then put skin in to soak)

Parsley

1 cup water

Preparation: Mix ginger root, lemon juice (and skin if you like), parsley, and 1 cup water. This becomes your concentrate. If you like, you can heat the concentrate until it boils, although it is not necessary to heat the concentrate. The concentrate will be very strong and is not intended as the cleanse. When you are ready to drink the cleanse, mix with eight ounces of soda water, water, and a touch of orange juice. The amount of concentrate will depend on your taste. Try mixing a small amount and test the taste. You can continue to add more if you would like. Then add agave or other recovery supersweetener to taste, but to a maximum of 1½ teaspoon.

You will love this cleanse and feel the benefits almost immediately. To save time, for this one I recommend preparing five cleanses at one time and storing them in the refrigerator. This is a great drink any time of the day. Add some seltzer and you have homemade ginger ale.

Exercise

I love this motto: "Move a muscle, change a thought." Living life as an isolated couch potato in a dark room will create a long-term hell for your body and put your recovery in jeopardy. Even small amounts of movement early on in your program can help to reduce cravings and the urge to use. Exercise will definitely contribute to improving your frame of mind.[240] If you work out in the morning, studies show you will benefit throughout the day.

It's simple: your body is designed to move. Movement is necessary for the flow of oxygenated blood to cells and to stimulate the production of hormones that ameliorate withdrawal symptoms and help to bridge the addict from withdrawal to recovery.[241] Substantial research has shown that exercise dramatically increases the chances of success in both short-term and long-term recovery, and in healing of both body and mind.[242,243] Aside from the physical effects of repairing damage to your body and vital organs, and encouraging regrowth of receptors in the brain,[244] exercise helps to reduce stress and anxiety. Since stress and anxiety are major underlying causes of urges to drink or use, by exercising you are effectively neutralizing addiction's hold over your mind.[245] Exercise is also a well-recognized tool for relapse prevention.[246]

Walk Three to Four Times a Day for Ten to Twenty Minutes

Study after study has shown the benefits of even small amounts of walking at a brisk pace, defined as the point at which it becomes difficult to talk comfortably due to increased breath rate, for ten minutes at a time.[247] So just start by walking ten minutes a day, and by day seven of your detox, get it up to twenty minutes. Walk to meetings, work, church, your lover's house, outpatient rehab, your therapist, the gym, or wherever. You can substitute bike riding as well; simply add 50 percent more time, fifteen to thirty minutes, and make sure you bike at a vigorous pace. This small amount of exercise churns up your metabolism, and you benefit in lots of other ways.

Your *metabolism* is defined as the number of calories burned by your body on a daily basis. Your *resting metabolism* is the amount of energy required for breathing, circulating blood, and maintaining body temperature. For most people, resting metabolism burns the most calories on a daily basis. Metabolism also includes calories burned through exercise. By exercising multiple times a day for short periods, you keep your metabolism going and elevated throughout the day. This helps stimulate production of natural hormones including dopamine and endorphins; burns fat and toxins; promotes the flow of fresh, oxygenated blood and water; and keeps you in a more positive mind-set throughout the day. Maintaining a more positive mind-set throughout the day can be difficult, but it's critical.

The average adult who walks briskly for ten to twenty minutes will see an increase in metabolic rate that usually lasts up to two or three hours.[248] Remember that for your pace to be considered brisk, you will need to feel challenged rather than comfortable. If your heart and body are not used to exercising, I do not suggest that you dramatically increase your heart rate without the advance knowledge and consent of your doctor.

By walking briskly when you wake up, again in the early afternoon, and then, if possible, in the late evening, you maximize the benefits all day long.

Check out Spiritual Adrenaline's recovery exercise page and blog on my website. There you will find core exercises you can do anywhere. You can jump-start the process of physical healing and the production of hormones and enzymes for the healing of your body, mind, and soul.

Yoga for Detox

Numerous yoga positions are designed to put pressure on your internal organs.[249] Each position is different and focuses on a specific organ. The pressure intentionally denies the organ fresh, oxygenated blood, and then when your body changes position, it floods the organ with fresh, oxygenated blood, cleansing the organ and assisting with the detox process. Achieving the correct position is critical to getting the intended benefits of each position.

The best part is that you don't have to do an hour or hour-and-a-half yoga class to get the benefits—although by all means do so if you want. Just practice these five positions, either one at a time or collectively, and you'll experience benefits.

I'm focusing here on five positions that you can do almost anywhere (except out on the street or in another such public setting). If you visit the exercise page at www.spiritualadrenaline.com, you can find these poses there. You can also locate them on the Spiritual Adrenaline Facebook page.

1. *Child's Pose:* This calms the nervous system and enhances blood flow to your lungs.

2. *Downward-Facing Dog:* With the heart higher than the head, fresh blood flows to your brain to help with circulation and calm the mind.

3. *Revolved Side Angle:* This flushes oxygen-rich blood through your torso, liver, kidneys, and pancreas, helping to remove toxins in the process.

4. *Half Lord of the Fishes:* This pose also courses oxygen-rich blood through the torso, liver, kidneys, and pancreas, helping to remove toxins.

5. *Legs Up Against the Wall:* This encourages the circulation of fresh, oxygenated blood through your liver and kidneys, assisting with detox. An additional benefit is that the position slows the nervous system, relieving stress.

Spirituality

Without faith in a power greater than yourself, it can be very difficult to achieve long-term recovery and, more importantly, happiness in recovery. *Eating right and exercise are spiritual tools.* Everything in this book can be a component of your spiritually based lifestyle. What greater spiritual experience can one ask for than taking care of one's body, the only one you will ever have, and bearing witness as your physical and mental health improves?

Some of these improvements you can see in the mirror, while others you cannot see but you can feel. Here are examples of a few simple inner improvements:

- Waking up excited about the day
- Appreciating rather than resenting the people around you; focusing on loving life rather than a substance
- Living with reduced fear, guilt, anxiety, and depression, and increased hope, empathy, patience, and love

Sure, it will take time, but right now in these seven days you are integrating the building blocks of a brighter future, in the context of both your recovery and your life.

Although this isn't the etymological basis, I suggest you think of the word *spiritual* as having two parts: spirit and ritual. Your spirit lies within you and simply needs to be awakened. Once awakened, your spirit will continue to grow. That's where the ritual comes in. I believe with all my heart that we must eat right and exercise regularly in order for our spirits to continue to remain fully awake. Only when we do these things over an extended period of time do they become a ritual and take on spiritual significance.

Bookend Workouts and Meetings

Now is the time to maximize your participation in your twelve-step program along with the benefits of the Spiritual Adrenaline lifestyle. If you are attending a morning meeting, you can bookend that meeting with a late-afternoon or evening workout. If you are attending a late-afternoon or evening meeting, you can bookend that meeting with a morning workout. By bookending your meetings and workouts at opposite ends of your day, you can stay in a recovery mind-set almost all day long. In between your meeting and workout, if you follow my nutritional recommendations you should have sustained fat-based energy throughout the day without spiking and then dropping your blood sugar. This will help decrease any urges and cravings.

The Importance of Your Spiritual Journal

Among the most important tools I recommend is your daily journal of your feelings, fears, concerns, regrets, guilty feelings, and aspirations and hopes for the future.

Don't say you'll do it when you get to it. Seize the day now! Don't say you'll start when you feel better; start today, and you'll feel better sooner!

Remember, the next time a company or a person peddles a pill, supplement, or other elixir as the solution to addiction, *get angry!* There isn't much money in sobriety, but there's lots of it in dealing with relapses. Rehabs and addiction recovery are a multibillion-dollar business that can only continue if you relapse and become perpetually sick. The tools Spiritual Adrenaline offers can help you break the cycle of active addiction, abstinence, and relapse, and help you find true sobriety and recovery in all aspects of your life.

Seven-Day Detox

Here's a plan for you to detox during the first seven days of following Spiritual Adrenaline. Do the same things every day for maximum results this week.

Morning

Nutrition:

- Morning cleanse with rotation between my recommended cleanses, and integrate foods from my recommended antioxidants, complex carbs and leafy greens into your breakfast.
- Integrate my recommended sweeteners in place of refined sugar. Here's my list:
  - Stevia
  - Raw honey
  - Truvia
  - Xylitol
- To cut back on caffeine, try my recommended alternatives to caffeinated coffee. Here's my list of options:
  - Decaf (still has 2 to 12 milligrams of caffeine)
  - Herbal coffee
  - Roasted grain beverage/Grain coffee
  - Yerba Mate
  - Matcha
  - Green tea
  - Herbal tea
  - Black tea
  - Chai latte

Exercise:

- Brisk morning walk of about fifteen to twenty minutes. This is a Zone 1 or 2–level workout.

Spiritual:

- Journal when you wake up about how you are feeling and your expectations for the day. If possible, create a gratitude list, and if you are feeling anxious or focused on resentments, journal about that. Try to be honest about what is causing these feelings inside you.

Late-Morning Snack

Pick a morning snack from my list of recommendations below.

- Greek yogurt with chocolate and berries
- Greek yogurt with fruit and wheat germ
- Cottage cheese with berries
- Low-sugar-content granola bar
- Toasted beet or sweet potato wedge with all-natural peanut butter

Midday

Nutrition:

- Midday cleanse with rotation between my recommended midday cleanses. During lunch, you are on your own. Avoid any processed or man-made carbs.

Exercise:

- Afternoon yoga detox stretch and/or brisk walk of about fifteen to twenty minutes. If possible, try to get out in nature for your afternoon exercise. Spend about three minutes on each of your yoga detox stretches. If you choose a brisk walk, keep it in Zone 1 or 2.

Spiritual:

- If you practice my recommended yoga detox stretch positions while taking deep breaths in and out, you should notice a change in your energy levels and how you feel.

Late-Afternoon Snack

- Pick a late-afternoon snack from my list of recommendations below.
  - Almonds, walnuts, macadamia nuts
  - Low-sugar-content granola bar
  - Avocado on whole-grain cracker or pita
  - All-natural peanut butter on whole-grain cracker or pita
  - Salad with veggies, nuts, berries, olive oil, and vinegar
  - Dark chocolate (small piece)
  - Hard-boiled egg
  - Veggie sticks (carrots, celery, etc.)
  - Toasted beet or sweet potato wedge (see recipes on our website). Add some all-natural peanut butter and it becomes totally yummy.
- Make sure to avoid caffeine and sugars after your late-afternoon snack. This will make it easier to sleep.

Evenings

Nutrition:

- Evening cleanse with rotation between our recommended evening cleanses, and integrate foods from my leafy greens, protein, and healthy fats into your dinner.
- Avoid caffeine and any sugars, natural or otherwise, at this time of the day. This will help you sleep.

Exercise:

- Evening brisk walk of about fifteen to twenty minutes. If you choose a brisk walk, keep it in Zone 1 or 2. If possible, try to get out in nature for your evening exercise. If possible, combine your evening workout with your spiritual program by walking to a meeting.

Spiritual:

- Twelve-step meeting (flexible based upon your schedule. If you need to go in the morning or midday, do so. Daily meeting attendance is highly recommended.)
- Write in your spiritual journal about your day. Take a look at your morning entry and see how you perceived the day and how

it actually turned out. If possible, draft another gratitude list with about five to ten items.

Late Night

Nutrition:

- Choose one of my late-night snacks if you get hungry or have cravings around bedtime or during the night. Many people get late-night cravings for carbs. My recommended foods have a small amount of carbs and are very filling. You may also want to add a teaspoon of MCT oil.

Exercise:

- If you are having trouble sleeping, try some of my yoga detox positions with deep breathing for about ten to fifteen minutes. This should help slow your mind down and make it easier to sleep.

Spiritual:

- If you are having trouble sleeping, try reading some recovery-focused literature. *Drop the Rock* and *The Ripple Effect* are highly recommended. Other options are the AA Big Book and *Twelve Steps and Twelve Traditions*.

Spiritual Adrenaline Inspiration: Rob A., Colorado

Rob Archuleta is a former crystal meth and ketamine ("Special K") addict who has double-digit recovery. He is the cofounder of Addict2Athlete, a program in Pueblo that integrates exercise and nutrition into the overall recovery of former athletes and addicts.

When I first got sober I gained a lot of weight; I went from 165 pounds to almost 250 in less than four months. My body was holding onto everything and the food tasted so good after not eating a normal meal for close to twelve years. Sober, I was also lost, as I had no direction. Drugs and alcohol had given me a purpose when I was using and drinking. Every day I woke up, started using, and had no direction except to get more drugs. Sober, I was bored. When I first started running, I had new purpose, a new direction, and when I was done there was always a feeling of accomplishment. I started to slowly take my life back, and the weight started falling off. Once I started to race, I was hooked; I had a new addiction. I erased the bad and started to replace it with good. My wife, who is also in recovery from crack, started to train with me, and we grew closer through the miles.

I love the Twelve Steps! They gave me my life back. I struggled with God; I had some traumatic childhood experiences, but when I was running and I would see a sunset, I knew there was a god, and I started to change. I started to believe, and on my runs I would reflect on the readings about recovery.

We all pick a drug that either fits our personalities or serves a purpose. I picked stimulants. I like to go fast, and I loved pushing the envelope. I need intensity in my life or I become self-destructive. I picked triathlons and CrossFit. Maybe someone who likes downers and alcohol more than I did would like yoga or tai chi. Do not do what everyone else does—*do you!*

CHAPTER THIRTEEN

The Spiritual Adrenaline Thirty-Day Program

The thirty-day program is a beginner's-level program that is suggested for you after you complete the seven-day detox. The thirty-day plan implements concepts from each of the main focus areas: nutrition, exercise, and spirituality.

In conjunction with this program, I recommend at least three twelve-step meetings a week. To really benefit and start to change how your mind works, I recommend a twelve-step meeting every day during the thirty days you follow this program. Remember, science now confirms that meeting attendance, step work, and following the other recommendations of twelve-step programs will impact your brain chemistry in a positive way. So make it your business to catch a meeting a day. Experiment with different meetings. Try a Y12SR meeting, Refuge Recovery, or a meditation meeting. The more you don't think you need a meeting, the more you probably do.

What Are Your Goals?
Rather than radically and drastically changing every aspect of your lifestyle, it's good to simply demonstrate your willingness to have an open mind and slowly incorporate lifestyle modifications into your day-to-day reality.

Research confirms that taking the process of change slowly and focusing on incremental and sustainable change over time dramatically increases the chances of long-term success.

Keep in mind that you do not need to plan to lose a huge amount of weight, run a marathon, or have a spiritual awakening of biblical proportions. Instead, you will look for subtle changes in how you perceive yourself, your environment, and others as a result of making a sincere effort to incorporate minor changes.

Nutrition

Weeks One and Two

In weeks one and two, there is minimal nutritional change from your present diet. You incorporate two evening dinners that are selected from a suggested menu. These foods are healthy protein and fat sources, along with a green vegetable, salad, and a healthy optional dessert. If you're not a "dessert person," you don't need to eat one. If you need a refresher on why you select these foods, reread the relevant sections of Chapter Three. Your late-night snack should also be selected from my list of healthy choices from Chapters Eight and Nine. For each meal you can also choose a recovery superspice from those listed in Chapters Eight and Nine. You can choose the spice based on your personal tastes or health history.

In the second week, you will add one day of a healthy breakfast along with a wholesome lunch. Your breakfast and lunch choices are designed to provide you with all the energy you will need from healthy fats, proteins, and carbohydrates. These foods will assist you in breaking the long-term reliance on sugars and caffeine for energy.

Weeks Three and Four

In weeks three and four, you will add an additional breakfast and lunch. This results in three days in a row with the equivalent of "nutritional medication." You should alternate your dinners, with at least one evening separating each. In weeks two and three, you should start to notice differences in your mood and energy on the days you follow the Spiritual Adrenaline program compared with those days when you are off program. These changes can be subtle and, for most people, take time. It's useful, however, to be conscious of these changes.

Exercise

Weeks One and Two

In weeks one and two, start with minimal exercise either at home, at a gym, or, even better, outside in nature. It's critical to set reasonable goals and achieve them rather than set yourself up for failure. Your exercise program therefore incorporates a brisk fifteen- to twenty-minute walk on one day during weeks one and two. If you are daring, you can turn your brisk walk into a walking meditation as I described in Chapter Eleven. In the second week, add in a second day of exercise. In week two, though, the second day of exercise is optional. Workouts in these weeks should be in Zone 1 or 2.

Weeks Three and Four

In weeks three and four you pick up the pace just a little more. You have a minimum of two days of cardiovascular exercise and one more day of weight training, yoga, or Pilates. However, it is important that your cardiovascular exercise happen on the same two days you incorporate your Spiritual Adrenaline dinner menu. This is important due to the interrelationships among your nutritional, physical, and spiritual self-care programs. Each enhances the benefits from the other. By incorporating exercise with meditation, then a healthy meal, you've provided your body with the much-needed nutrients for mind, body, and soul. Throw in a meeting and you will feel amazing. Workouts in these weeks should be in Zone 1, 2, or 3.

Spirituality

You'll notice the Spiritual Adrenaline thirty-day plan has a lot of repetition. It's the repetition of certain tasks and actions while being mindful that it makes something simple, such as food preparation, into a ritual, and later, a spiritual tool. Keep in mind that the redundancy in this thirty-day plan is by design, not accident.

Weeks One and Two

In weeks one and two, ease into the spirituality aspect of the program. One of the fundamental premises of Spiritual Adrenaline is that it is incredibly difficult to connect with spirituality when your body is not healthy. That's why you should focus on nutrition and exercise in the early stages and then gradually introduce spiritual concepts. If you've incorporated a walking meditation into your brisk walk, you've already integrated a spiritual practice into your day.

A second spiritual practice will be to purchase food and prepare your two evening meals during the week. Some may say this is silly and not a spiritual practice, but I disagree. As I explain in Chapter Eleven, the foods you choose to purchase and eat are among the most important choices you make in your life. Food contains substances, and when you eat, you are putting those substances into your body—*the only body you will ever have.* Just as you must think about what substances are introduced into your body in the context of alcohol and other drugs, you should apply that same mindfulness to food.

A third spiritual practice is preparing your food. Again, food contains substances, and you will be putting those substances into your body. You want to think about that as you prepare your food, and thank yourself for taking the time to prepare foods that will nourish your body and mind rather than hurt it. Enjoy the process, as food preparation is basic self-care and an important tool to develop early in the recovery process. After dinner you are free to do whatever you normally do. A twelve-step meeting is highly recommended.

A fourth spiritual practice is my recommendation to turn off your cell phone from approximately 9:00 p.m. until after your morning meditation program the next day. I recommend one overnight a week in the first week and adding a second overnight in the second week. If you need a refresher on why this is such a powerful spiritual tool, reread the relevant sections of Chapter Eleven. You can use the time in the evening when you are truly alone, with no external interference, to journal, read recovery literature, conduct a Tenth Step inventory, and more, as long as the focus is on things that will enhance your spiritual journey.

A fifth spiritual practice is journaling during your morning meditation on at least two mornings a week. Journaling can be done after you shut down your cell phone at night, and/or the following morning as part of your self-care program. For a refresher on the importance of journaling, review Chapters Six, Seven, and Eleven.

Weeks Three and Four

In weeks three and four, continue all of the spiritual tools you implemented in weeks one and two: walking meditation; food purchasing; food preparation; shutting your cell phone off one night during week one, and then two nights during week two; engaging in a morning meditative practice at least two mornings a week; at the very least two twelve-step meetings a week; and journaling. That is a lot of spiritual tools!

In weeks three and four, add in one more nuance. Go back at some point and review your journals from your seven-day detox and weeks one and two to identify how you felt then and how you feel now, and note any changes. Review your earlier journals at least once or twice a week as you are moving forward or when you are feeling frustrated about continuing with the program. Hopefully, when implementing the tools consistently for more than fourteen days, you should start to notice subtle changes in your thoughts and mood. By reviewing your early journals and comparing your past journals to your present reality, you will be able to identify the positive changes that are happening. Acknowledging the positive changes and giving yourself credit for the hard work you put in will keep you motivated to keep going.

Thirty-Day Spiritual Adrenaline Program
Nutrition

Review my recovery superfoods. I have a large number of options to ensure that you are not eating the same old thing every day. During your seven-day detox, I have kept the choices minimal to make it easier to purchase the foods you need and to make preparation simple. I now change things up quite a bit. With so many choices, make sure to vary what you are eating, as each one of the superfoods packs a different nutritional punch. Some may look alike, but the similarities end there. If you need a refresher on the nutrients in each and the benefits you derive from eating them, head back to the Addiction Paleo chapter.

I suggest combinations of recovery superfoods for the maximum nutritional benefit. If you decide to go outside my recommendations, make sure you know the macronutrients in the foods and, to the extent possible, ensure the foods are consistent with my recommendations.

If you are counting calories and macros, I recommend that of all daily calories, 50 percent should be from fat, 30 percent from protein, and 20 percent from carbohydrates. To determine the number of calories you should be taking in every day, the simple method is to add a zero to your weight.

If you want to save yourself a lot of time, try the carb cutoff method instead. Set a carb cutoff time of late afternoon or early evening. Then, remember to eat to be FAB: for **F**uel early in the day, to remain **A**ctive at midday, and then to **B**uild into the evening and overnight. Front-load your carbs into your breakfast, midmorning snack, and lunch. Thereafter, cut back until your cutoff time. Given that it's difficult to completely cut out carbs, I offer several filling, low-carb late-night snacks to help take the edge off.

Vegetables

- Asparagus
- Beets
- Broccoli
- Carrots
- Cauliflower
- Collard greens
- Garlic
- Green peas
- Kale
- Mushrooms
- Parsley
- Spinach
- Sweet potato
- Tomatoes
- Watercress

Fruits

- Apple
- Blueberries
- Cantaloupe
- Cranberries
- Goji berries
- Grapefruit
- Kiwi
- Lemon
- Papaya
- Pomegranate
- Pumpkin
- Raspberries
- Strawberries
- Watermelon

Seeds, Nuts, and Beans

- Almonds
- Black beans
- Cashews
- Chia seeds
- Chickpeas
- Flaxseed

- Fennel
- Garbanzo beans
- Lentils
- Pecans
- Pistachios

- Peanuts
- Pumpkin seeds
- Sunflower seeds
- Wheat germ
- Walnuts

Protein Sources

- Fish
- Grass-fed meat
- Turkey
- Oily fish (salmon, for example)

- Nonoily fish (cod, bass, etc.)
- Soybeans
- Eggs

Carbs

- Brown rice
- Quinoa
- Whole-grain bread

- Ezekiel bread (sprout based)
- Tapioca bread
- Coconut bread

Cooking Oil/Spreads

- Coconut oil

- Extra virgin olive oil

Beverages

- Green tea
- Dandelion tea
- Matcha

- Light-roast coffee
- Water

Condiments

- Sea salt
- Black pepper
- Vegetable ketchup

- Dijon mustard
- Spicy mustard
- Hot sauce

Chocolate

- Cocoa content of 70 percent or more

Recovery Superspices
- Turmeric (curcumin)
- Ginger
- Cinnamon
- Berberine
- Cumin
- Garlic
- Nutmeg
- Paprika
- Vanilla flavor (alcohol free)

Sweeteners
- Stevia
- Raw honey
- Truvia
- Date sugar
- Xylitol
- Swerve

Baking Alternatives
- Tapioca starch
- Coconut starch

Midmorning Snack
- Flaxseed muffin with fruit and nuts
- Three-bean salad with extra virgin olive oil
- Apple, orange, grapes
- Sweet potato brownie
- Greek yogurt with chocolate and berries
- Greek yogurt with fruit and wheat germ
- Cottage cheese with berries
- Low-sugar-content granola bar
- Toasted beet or sweet potato wedge

Midafternoon Snack
- Almonds, walnuts, macadamia nuts
- Low-sugar-content granola bar
- Avocado on whole-grain cracker or pita
- All-natural peanut butter on whole-grain cracker or pita
- Salad with veggies, nuts, berries, olive oil, and vinegar
- Dark chocolate (small piece)
- Hard-boiled egg
- Veggie sticks (carrots, celery, etc.)
- Toasted beet or sweet potato wedge with all-natural peanut butter
- Keto chili

Late-Night Snack
- Rice cakes
- Ezekiel bread
- Casein protein
- Frozen blueberries
- Multigrain pretzels
- Popcorn
- Unsalted almonds
- Liquid egg white with veggies

Suggested Breakfasts
- Omelet (either egg white or whole egg); mix in vegetables of your choosing and choice of condiment
- Turkey bacon
- Granola or flax, wheat germ, chia seeds, sunflower seeds, fruits, honey or other sweetener
- Cottage cheese with seeds, nuts, berries, honey or other sweetener
- Steel-cut oatmeal with all-natural peanut butter, berries, and cinnamon or other superspices
- Boiled eggs, spinach or kale, and avocado spread on whole-wheat or multigrain bread
- Protein pancakes with fruit of your choosing and honey, spinach or kale, whole-wheat toast with all-natural peanut butter
- Sweet potato pancakes with fruit of your choosing and honey, spinach or kale, whole-wheat toast with all-natural peanut butter
- Milk and honey chilled overnight with chia
- Blueberry or banana chilled overnight with flax

Suggested Lunch Meals
- Fresh turkey, chicken, or ham on wheat or whole-grain bread; watercress, tomato, onion, or other vegetables; condiments of your choosing
- Three-bean salad with extra virgin olive oil; parsley, tomato, onion (can easily be turned into three-bean chili), with whole-wheat or whole-grain bread
- Grass-fed sirloin burger on whole-wheat pita; onions, vegetable ketchup or other condiments
- Turkey or veggie burger on whole-grain pita or without bread; salad with veggies of your choosing

- Chicken breast, turkey bacon, avocado salad
  - Chicken breast or salmon/sea bass; walnut, strawberry, and pistachio salad

Suggested Dinners
  - Sea bass (4 to 6 oz.), asparagus, salad with veggies of your choosing, baked sweet potato (3 to 4 oz.) or sweet potato fries, balsamic vinaigrette or other low- or no-fat dressing, healthy dessert
  - Salmon (4 to 6 oz.), spinach, salad with veggies of your choosing, baked sweet potato (3 to 4 oz.) or sweet potato fries, balsamic vinaigrette or other low- or no-fat dressing
  - Baked chicken breast, sea bass, or salmon with tomato, parsley, onion, and superspices
  - Sirloin (80 to 90 percent lean)
  - Oven-roasted chicken breast with superspices
  - Grass-fed sirloin burger on whole-wheat pita, onions, vegetable ketchup or other condiments
  - Turkey tacos
  - Stuffed peppers
  - Chicken vegetable soup

Suggested Desserts
I recommend checking out www.EXPNutrition.com for some healthy and delicious dessert recommendations from Melanie Albert. Here are a couple of my own:
  - Flourless chocolate cupcakes with nuts and fruit
  - Sweet potato pie
  - Flaxseed muffins

Suggested Detox Drinks
  - Fresh detox ginger ale
  - Cinnamon, nutmeg
  - Cumin, lemon, fennel
  - Turmeric, garlic, almond

Exercise

During the seven-day detox program, I include brisk walks, preferably in nature, to get you up and moving. For many, it may have been years since they engaged in any activity because of their disease. We all start from different places, but if we stay committed, over time we progress and things get easier and more fun. Remember, life begins outside your comfort zone. So let's go there.

Here are my recommended exercise tools:

- Bookend your meetings with workouts to maximize the benefits.
- When possible, try to exercise in nature.
- Turn your workouts into meditations.
- Time your nutrients to achieve your goals.
- Utilize Fitbit and other technology to your benefit.
- Remember cardio Zones 1, 2, 3, and 4.

Spiritual

Hopefully after detoxing, you are starting to feel better physically and emotionally. The Spiritual Adrenaline spiritual tools integrate mind, body, and spirit recovery. Although you are free to implement any spiritual tools that you feel comfortable with, my recommendations are intended to cross over between different areas of focus. For example, if you can turn your meal preparation and cleanup into a meditation, you are saving time and doubling the benefit.

Here are my recommended spiritual tools (see Chapter Eleven):

- Airplane mode
- Mealtime meditations
- Exercise meditations
- Full-body meditations
- Green fellowship
- "How It Works" meditation
- Supreme teacher
- Naps
- Music
- Gratitude trips
- Reading

Day-to-Day Guide

Day One

This is the day to set your baseline, journal about why you are trying this program, and set down your aspirations for the future. When you started the seven-day detox, you should have chosen whatever external and internal metrics made sense for you. It's too early to expect any change; you will measure those again in a couple of weeks. However, if you haven't yet set your day-one metrics, now is the time. As a reminder, here they are again:

- *Internal Measures (based upon your blood work):* white blood cell count, triglycerides, sodium, blood sugar, good cholesterol, bad cholesterol, cortisol, BUN levels, creatinine serum, ALT and AST levels, albumin, alkaline phosphatase, bilirubin, and testosterone-free levels. You can also use your blood pressure as an internal measure. If you are a smoker, you may want to have your lung capacity tested as well while smoking and then after you quit.
- *External Measures:* "before" and "after" photos, muscle measurements, weight, and body fat. Remember, BMI, or body mass index, is not recommended.
- Make time to write out a gratitude list and conduct a Tenth Step inventory. Although we take things one day at a time, you want to maximize your chances of success. Make sure that over the next twenty-nine days you have no urgent matters to attend to, and to the extent you can lighten your load to focus on this program, try to do so.

Day Two

Nutrition:

- The food you purchase today will be your dinner tomorrow evening. The choice of where you go to shop for your meal is important. Try to get the freshest veggies possible at a farmer's market, and antibiotic/hormone-free meats, chicken, and/or fish. This is all going into your body, so let's be really choosy. If you are vegetarian or vegan, you can use an alternative protein source such as soybeans, nuts, or green veggies.

- If you're ambitious, rather than doing just one dinner this week, you can try for two. If you are going to cook two, I recommend a one-day separation between meals.
- Your carb cutoff should be at about 6:00 or 7:00 p.m. at the latest.
- If you choose to have a late-night snack, choose from among my recommendations.

Exercise:
- Make sure to take a brisk walk today of about fifteen to twenty minutes. If possible, walk in nature or a green setting.
- If you are tracking your heart rate, keep your workouts in week one in Zone 1. However, progressively increase the intensity of your walk or other activity to challenge yourself.

Spirituality:
- Start your day by writing in your spiritual journal and integrating other morning self-care-based practices into your morning routine. Here are some recommendations:
  - Make your bed
  - Meditation
  - Read recovery literature
  - Full-body meditation
- You may also choose to prepare your food this evening and turn that preparation into a spiritual practice. You do this by shutting off your electronic devices and focusing on what you are buying, the ingredients in what you are buying, and how specific foods can either enhance or undercut your recovery.
- Attend a twelve-step meeting and, to the extent possible, bookend it with your brisk walk.

Day Three

Nutrition:
- The food you purchased yesterday is dinner tonight. While preparing your dinner, make sure to practice my recommended meditations as you prepare your food and then eat. While eating your dinner, also integrate my recommended meditation.

- Make sure to use at least one of our recovery superspices with your dinner tonight.
- Keep your carb cutoff at 6:00 to 7:00 p.m. all of this week.
- If you choose to have a late-night snack today, choose from among my recommendations.

Exercise:
- Make sure to take a brisk walk today of about fifteen to twenty minutes. If possible, walk in nature or a green setting.
- If you are tracking your heart rate, keep your workouts in week one in Zone 1. However, progressively increase the intensity of your walk or other activity to challenge yourself.

Spirituality:
- Start your day by writing in your spiritual journal and integrating other morning self-care-based practices. Here are some recommendations:
  - Make your bed
  - Meditation
  - Read recovery literature
  - Full-body meditation
- After dinner, wash the dishes; make sure electronic devices are off. Be present and really focus on cleaning the dishes and putting them out to dry.
- Attend a twelve-step meeting and, to the extent possible, bookend it with your brisk walk.
- Shut off your electronic devices about an hour before you go to bed. Leave those devices off all night.

Day Four

Nutrition:
- Just like on day two, purchase food today for your dinner tomorrow evening. This second dinner is optional but recommended. The choice of where you go to shop for your meal is important. Also, vary the menu from what you had for dinner earlier in the week. For example, if you had an oily fish like salmon, tonight have a lean steak or free–range, antibiotic-free chicken. If you are vegetarian or

vegan, you can use an alternative protein source such as beans, nuts, or green veggies.

- Carb cutoff remains at 6:00 to 7:00 p.m.
- If you choose not to purchase food today, you're on your own for the day. However, if you choose to have a late-night snack, choose from among my recommendations.

Exercise:

- Make sure to take a brisk walk today of about fifteen to twenty minutes. If possible, walk in nature or a green setting.
- If you are tracking your heart rate, keep your workouts in week one in Zone 1. However, progressively increase the intensity of your walk or other activity to challenge yourself.

Spirituality:

- This morning, your electronic devices should be off when you wake up. Enjoy the solitude and journal about how you may feel different waking up this way. I recommend you start your day with writing in your spiritual journal and integrating other morning self-care-based practices. Here are some recommendations:
  - Make your bed
  - Meditation
  - Read recovery literature
  - Full-body meditation
- Attend a twelve-step meeting and, to the extent possible, bookend it with a brisk walk.

Day Five

- Repeat what you did on day three.
- If you are preparing and eating the optional second dinner tonight, make sure to integrate my recommended meditations for meal preparation and at dinner time. Also use at least one of my recovery superspices, and if possible, more than one.

Day Six

Nutrition:

- You are off today and can eat whatever you like. However, when eating, be mindful of the substances that compose the foods and how you feel after you eat them.

Exercise:

- Make sure to take a brisk walk today of about fifteen to twenty minutes. If possible, walk in nature or a green setting.
- If you are tracking your heart rate, keep your workouts in week one in Zone 1. However, progressively increase the intensity of your walk or other activity to challenge yourself.

Spirituality:

- Make sure to write in your spiritual journal in the morning when you wake up. Follow the morning self-care regime you practiced earlier in the week or vary it a little. You may want to try each of my recommendations to see which one works best for you.
- Today make sure to journal about what you are eating given that you are on your own today.
  - Do you feel guilty about what you are eating?
  - Are you embarrassed about what you are eating?
  - How do you feel after eating these foods?
  - Do you feel better or worse after eating these foods than you did when you prepared your dinners this week?
  - Did you enjoy purchasing foods for dinner this week?
  - Did you enjoy preparing those foods?

Days Seven and Eight

You're off. Enjoy your weekend. The only optional activity is to purchase food for the week ahead. Next week, you'll be preparing two morning breakfasts and two lunches. So you have more food to buy. If you are tight on time during the week, it's highly recommended to get your food shopping done on these days. It's also highly recommended that you put time aside to journal. Some recommendations on topics for your journal are:

- What worked well?

- What didn't?
- What do you want to try differently?
- How was your lifestyle last week different from the past?
- How do you feel during your morning self-care program, when shopping for food, during your brisk walk, and while preparing or eating your home-cooked meals?
- What are your aspirations for next week?
- Move your carb cutoff to 5:00 or 6:00 p.m. this week.

Congratulations on completing week one. Now let's get focused on week two.

Day Nine

Nutrition:

- The food you purchase today or on your days off will be for two breakfasts, two lunches, and two dinners. The choice of where you go to shop for your meal is important. If possible, try to get to a farmer's market and a place where you can buy the freshest meat, poultry, or fish.
- This morning, after your morning self-care program, you will prepare breakfast. Review my recovery superfoods and include some that you like in your breakfast menu. There are recipes in the back of this book that you can follow, or you can create your own.
- Include with your breakfast as many recovery superspices as possible.
- You should also prepare and pack your lunch for today. Go over the same recovery superfoods I covered for breakfast and check out the full list to help you plan your lunch. Try to incorporate my recommended superspices into your lunch menu as well. If you need help, check out my lunch suggestions.
- Remember that you are beginning to transition away from carbohydrates after lunch and should start to focus on taking more protein and fat and fewer carbs. With this in mind, you can prepare your lunch.
- Your carb cutoff this week should be 5:00 to 6:00 p.m.
- If you choose to have a late-night snack, choose from among my recommendations. I recommend staying away from carbs after the late afternoon. However, if you are craving carbohydrates in the

evening or before going to sleep, pick from my recommendations that either have no carbs or are low in carbs and very filling. They should help you get through it if you are craving carbs. If you are still craving carbs, have a teaspoon of MCT oil and that should calm your brain down.

Exercise:
- Make sure to take a brisk walk today of about fifteen to twenty minutes. If possible, walk in nature or a green setting.
- If you are tracking your heart rate, keep your workouts in Zone 2. However, progressively increase the intensity of your walk or other activity to challenge yourself.

Spirituality:
- Start your day by writing in your spiritual journal and integrating other morning self-care-based practices. Here are some recommendations:
  - Meditation
  - Read recovery literature
  - Full-body meditation
- You may also choose to prepare your food this evening for tomorrow's dinner and turn your meal preparation into a spiritual practice. You do this by shutting off your electronic devices and focusing on what you are buying, the ingredients in what you are buying, and how specific foods can either enhance or undercut your recovery.
- Attend a twelve-step meeting and, to the extent possible, bookend it with your brisk walk.

Day Ten

Nutrition:
- The food you purchased yesterday is dinner tonight. While preparing your dinner, make sure to practice my recommended meditation. While eating your dinner, also integrate my recommended meditations.
- Make sure to use at least one of my recovery superspices with your dinner tonight.
- Your carb cutoff this week should be 5:00 to 6:00 p.m.

- If you choose to have a late-night snack, choose from among my recommendations. I recommend staying away from carbs after the late afternoon. However, if you are craving carbohydrates in the evening or before going to sleep, pick from my recommendations that either have no carbs or are low in carbs and very filling. They should help you get through carb cravings. If you are still craving carbs, have a teaspoon of MCT oil and that should calm your brain down.

Exercise:
- Make sure to take a brisk walk today of about fifteen to twenty minutes. If possible, walk in nature or a green setting.
- If you are tracking your heart rate, keep your workouts in week one in Zone 2. However, progressively increase the intensity of your walk or other activity to challenge yourself.

Spirituality:
- Start your day by writing in your spiritual journal and integrating other morning self-care-based practices. Here are some recommendations:
  - Make your bed
  - Meditation
  - Read recovery literature
  - Full-body meditation
- Attend a twelve-step meeting and, to the extent possible, bookend it with your brisk walk.

Day Eleven

Nutrition:
- Follow the same nutritional regimen as you did on day nine. Today you will be preparing your breakfast and lunch. Utilize my recommended meditations while preparing these meals. Also, after preparing your meals, check to see what items you may be running low on or out of. Later this evening, you can shop for whatever you need for the rest of the week.

- If you go food shopping, remember to integrate my recommended meditation, turning electronic devices off and focusing on the foods you are buying.
- Your carb cutoff is 5:00 to 6:00 p.m. this week.
- If you choose to have a late-night snack, choose from among my recommendations. I recommend staying away from carbs after the late afternoon. However, if you are craving carbohydrates in the evening or before going to sleep, pick from my recommendations that either have no carbs or are low in carbs and very filling. They should help you get through carb cravings. If you are still craving carbs, have a teaspoon of MCT oil and that should calm down your brain.

Exercise:
- Make sure to take a brisk walk today of about fifteen to twenty minutes. If you are feeling up to it, extend the time frame to twenty to thirty minutes or beyond. If possible, walk in nature or a green setting.
- If you are tracking your heart rate, keep your workouts in week one in Zone 2. However, progressively increase the intensity of your walk or other activity to challenge yourself.

Spirituality:
- Start your day by writing in your spiritual journal and integrating other morning self-care-based practices. Here are some recommendations:
  - Make your bed
  - Meditation
  - Full-body meditation
  - Read recovery literature
- Turn off your cell phone and other electronic devices about one hour before going to bed tonight. Leave those devices off all night.

Day Twelve

Nutrition:
- Follow the same nutritional regimen as you did on day ten. Today you will be preparing your dinner. Utilize my recommended

meditations while preparing your dinner. Make sure to include at least one of my recovery superspices with your dinner.

- The carb cutoff remains at 5:00 to 6:00 p.m.
- If you choose to have a late-night snack, choose from among my recommendations. I recommend staying away from carbs after the late afternoon. However, if you are craving carbohydrates in the evening or before going to sleep, pick from my recommendations that either have no carbs or are low in carbs and very filling. They should help you get through it if you are craving carbs. If you are still craving carbs, have a teaspoon of MCT oil and that should calm your brain down.

Exercise:

- Make sure to take a brisk walk today of about fifteen to twenty minutes. If you are feeling up to it, extend the time frame to twenty to thirty minutes or beyond. If possible, walk in nature or a green setting.
- If you are tracking your heart rate, keep your workouts in week one in Zone 2. However, progressively increase the intensity of your walk or other activity to challenge yourself.

Spirituality:

- Start your day by writing in your spiritual journal and integrating other morning self-care-based practices. Here are some recommendations:
  - Make your bed
  - Meditation
  - Full-body meditation
  - Read recovery literature
- Turn on your cell phone and other electronic devices after your morning self-care-based program.
- Attend a twelve-step meeting and bookend it to the extent possible with your brisk walk.

Day Thirteen

Nutrition:

- The only meal you will be preparing today is your lunch. Follow the same protocols that you did on days nine and eleven for the preparation of your lunch. (On those days you also prepared breakfast. You are free to add your breakfast today, but it's optional.) Make sure to include at least one of my recovery superspices in your lunch.
- The carb cutoff for this week remains at 5:00 to 6:00 p.m.
- If you choose to have a late-night snack, choose from among my recommendations. I recommend staying away from carbs after the late afternoon. However, if you are craving carbohydrates in the evening or before going to sleep, pick from my late-night snack recommendations that either have no carbs or are low in carbs and very filling. They should help you get through it if you are craving carbs. If you are still craving carbs, have a teaspoon of MCT oil and that should calm down your brain.

Exercise:

- Make sure to take a brisk walk today of about fifteen to twenty minutes. If you are feeling up to it, extend the time frame to twenty to thirty minutes or beyond. If possible, walk in nature or a green setting.
- If you are tracking your heart rate, keep your workouts in week one in Zone 2. However, progressively increase the intensity of your walk or other activity to challenge yourself.

Spirituality:

- Start your day by writing in your spiritual journal and integrating other morning self-care-based practices. Here are some recommendations:
  - Make your bed
  - Meditation
  - Full-body meditation
  - Read recovery literature
- Attend a twelve-step meeting and bookend it to the extent possible with your brisk walk.

Days Fourteen and Fifteen

You're off. Enjoy your weekend. There are three recommended activities for this weekend. First, purchase food for the week ahead. In week three, you'll be preparing two breakfasts, two lunches, and two dinners. You want to also make sure to have healthy snacks for during the day and your late-night snack, if needed. If you are tight on time during the week, it's highly recommended that you purchase your food over the weekend.

Second, this week we begin to integrate more rigorous physical exercise. You may decide to integrate weight training, yoga, Pilates, CrossFit, or some other form of exercise. My recommendations are just that, recommendations. You do you! My only suggestion is that you ensure you have whatever clothes or equipment you will need to participate.

Third, just like last week, it's also highly recommended that you put time aside time to journal. Some recommendations on topics for your journal are:

- What worked well?
- What didn't?
- What do you want to try differently?
- How was your lifestyle last week different from the past?
- How do you feel during your morning self-care program, when shopping for food, during your brisk walk, and while preparing or eating your home-cooked meals?
- What are your aspirations for next week?

You are halfway through! Let's enjoy the weekend and get pumped for the final two weeks.

Day Sixteen

Nutrition:

- Prepare your breakfast and lunch today. Make sure to integrate my recovery superspices into both meals.
- Make sure to pack your midmorning and midafternoon snacks. If you need help with ideas, check out my food list.
- Your carb cutoff should be around 5:00 p.m. this week.

- This evening you purchase and/or begin to prepare your dinners for later in the week. Make sure to integrate my mindfulness meditations while purchasing, preparing, and eating your meals all week.
- If you choose to have a late-night snack, choose from my list of recommended late-night snacks. If you are still craving carbs, have a teaspoon of MCT oil and that should calm down your brain.

Exercise:

- Make sure to take a brisk walk today of about fifteen to twenty minutes. If you are feeling up to it, extend the time frame to twenty to thirty minutes or beyond. If possible, walk in nature or a green setting.
- If you are tracking your heart rate, keep your workouts in Zones 2 and 3. However, progressively increase the intensity of your walk or other activity to challenge yourself. If you are still in a Zone 1 range, take your time and progress at the pace that is appropriate for you.

Spirituality:

- Start your day with writing in your spiritual journal and integrating other morning self-care-based practices from my list of recommendations.
- Attend a twelve-step meeting and bookend it to the extent possible with your brisk walk.

Day Seventeen

Nutrition:

- Prepare your dinner tonight with my recovery superspices integrated into your dinner. While preparing and eating your meal and cleaning up, I recommend that you practice my mindfulness meditations.
- Make sure to pack your midmorning and midafternoon snacks. If you need help with ideas, check out my list.
- Your carb cutoff should be around 5:00 p.m. this week.
- If you choose to have a late-night snack, choose from my list of recommended late-night snacks. If you are still craving carbs, have a teaspoon of MCT oil and that should calm down your brain.

Exercise:

- This morning you integrate a group activity, preferably in the morning after your morning self-care program. Pick an activity that you enjoy and go for it. Don't let your critical parent and stinking thinking keep you from going. Ninety percent of the challenge is getting there.
- If you are tracking your heart rate, keep your workouts in Zones 2 and 3. However, progressively increase the intensity of your walk or other activity to challenge yourself. If you are still in a Zone 1 range, take your time and progress at the pace that is appropriate for you.
- Keep your brisk walk in your routine today. If you work out in the morning, try to take your brisk walk in the later afternoon. If you need to work out in the later afternoon or evening, try to move your brisk walk to morning. If you are feeling up to it, extend the time frame to twenty to thirty minutes or beyond. If possible, walk in nature or a green setting.

Spirituality:

- Start your day by writing in your spiritual journal and integrating other morning self-care-based practices from our list of recommendations.
- Attend a twelve-step meeting and bookend it to the extent possible with your group activity.

Day Eighteen

Nutrition:

- Follow the same protocols that you did on day sixteen by preparing breakfast and lunch today. Make sure to integrate my recovery superspices into both meals.
- Make sure to pack your midmorning and midafternoon snacks. If you need help with ideas, check out my list.
- Your carb cutoff should be around 5:00 p.m. this week.
- This evening you purchase and/or begin to prepare your dinners for later in the week. Make sure to integrate my mindfulness meditations while purchasing, preparing, and eating your meals all week.

- If you choose to have a late-night snack, choose from my list of recommendations. If you are still craving carbs, have a teaspoon of MCT oil and that should calm down your brain.

Exercise:
- Make sure to take a brisk walk today of about fifteen to twenty minutes. If you are feeling up to it, extend the time frame to twenty to thirty minutes or beyond. If possible, walk in nature or a green setting. If you are feeling ambitious, add a second brisk walk into your day today.
- If you are tracking your heart rate, keep your workouts in Zones 2 and 3. However, progressively increase the intensity of your walk or other activity to challenge yourself. If you are still in a Zone 1 range, take your time and progress at the pace that is appropriate for you.

Spirituality:
- Start your day by writing in your spiritual journal and integrating other morning self-care-based practices from my list of recommendations.
- Attend a twelve-step meeting and bookend it to the extent possible with your brisk walk.
- Turn off your cell phone and other electronic devices tonight about an hour before you go to bed.

Day Nineteen

Nutrition:
- Prepare your dinner tonight with my recovery superspices integrated into your dinner. While preparing and eating your meal and cleaning up, I recommend you practice my mindfulness meditations.
- Make sure to pack your midmorning and midafternoon snacks. If you need help with ideas, check out my list.
- Your carb cutoff should be around 5:00 p.m. this week.
- If you choose to have a late-night snack, choose from my list of recommended late-night snacks. If you are still craving carbs, have a teaspoon of MCT oil and that should calm down your brain.

Exercise:

- This morning you again integrate a group activity, preferably in the morning after our morning self-care program. Pick an activity that you enjoy and go for it.
- If you are tracking your heart rate, keep your workouts in week one in Zones 2 and 3. However, progressively increase the intensity of your walk or other activity to challenge yourself. If you are still in a Zone 1 range, take your time and progress at the pace that is appropriate for you.
- Keep your brisk walk in your routine today. If you work out in the morning, try to take your brisk walk in the later afternoon. If you need to work out in the later afternoon or evening, try to move your brisk walk to morning. If you are feeling up to it, extend the time frame to twenty to thirty minutes or beyond. If possible, walk in nature or a green setting.

Spirituality:

- Start your day with writing in your spiritual journal and integrating other morning self-care-based practices from my list of recommendations.
- After your morning self-care program, turn on your cell phone and other electronic devices.
- Attend a twelve-step meeting and bookend it to the extent possible with your group activity.

Day Twenty

Nutrition:

- Prepare your lunch for today and integrate my recovery superspices. While preparing and eating your meal and cleaning up, I recommend you practice our mindfulness meditations.
- Make sure to pack your midmorning and midafternoon snacks. If you need help with ideas, check out our list.
- Your carb cutoff should be around 5:00 p.m. this week.
- If you choose to have a late-night snack, choose from my list of recommended late-night snacks.

Exercise:

- Keep your brisk walk in your routine today. If you are feeling up to it, extend the time frame to twenty to thirty minutes or beyond or add a second brisk walk at some point during the day. If possible, walk in nature or a green setting.
- If you are tracking your heart rate, keep your workouts in week one in Zones 2 and 3. However, progressively increase the intensity of your walk or other activity to challenge yourself. If you are still in a Zone 1 range, take your time and progress at the pace that is appropriate for you.

Spirituality:

- Start your day with writing in your spiritual journal and integrating other morning self-care-based practices from my list of recommendations.
- Attend a twelve-step meeting and bookend it to the extent possible with your group activity.

Days Twenty-One and Twenty-Two

You're off. Enjoy your weekend. There are three recommended activities for this weekend. Those recommendations are the same as the ones for last weekend.

First, purchase food for the week ahead. In week four you'll prepare three breakfasts, three lunches, and three dinners. This means you will need to plan and think ahead. You want to also make sure to have healthy snacks for during the day and for your late-night snack, if needed. If you are tight on time during the week, it's highly recommended that you purchase your food over the weekend.

Second, this week you integrate three morning workouts. Again, you choose the activity that is most appealing to you.

Third, just like last week, it's also highly recommended that you put time aside to journal. Some recommendations on topics for your journal are:

- What worked well?
- What didn't?
- What do you want to try differently?
- How was your lifestyle last week different from the past?

- How do you feel during your morning self-care program when shopping for food, during your brisk walk, and while preparing or eating your home-cooked meals?
- What are your aspirations for next week?

You're almost there! Enjoy the weekend and get pumped for the final week.

Day Twenty-Three

Nutrition:

- Prepare your breakfast and lunch today. Make sure to integrate recovery superspices into both meals.
- Make sure to pack your midmorning and midafternoon snacks. If you need help with ideas, check out my list.
- Your carb cutoff should be around 5:00 p.m. this week.
- This evening you purchase and/or begin to prepare your dinners for later in the week. Make sure to integrate my mindfulness meditations while purchasing, preparing, and eating your meals all week.
- If you choose to have a late-night snack, choose from my list of recommended late-night snacks. If you are still craving carbs, have a teaspoon of MCT oil. That should calm down your brain.

Exercise:

- This morning I include a group activity/workout of your choosing. If you cannot work out in the morning, then move this activity to late afternoon or early evening. Try to the extent possible to bookend this workout with your daily brisk walk.
- Make sure to take a brisk walk today of about fifteen to twenty minutes. If you are feeling up to it, extend the time frame to twenty to thirty minutes or beyond. If possible, walk in nature or a green setting.
- If you are tracking your heart rate, keep your workouts in Zones 2 and 3 and, if you are comfortable doing so, challenge yourself to take it up to Zone 4 intermittently. However, go with what you feel is best for you, and make sure to keep your zone appropriate for your age, health, and ability.

Spirituality:

- Start your day by writing in your spiritual journal and integrating other morning self-care-based practices from my list of recommendations.
- Attend a twelve-step meeting and bookend it to the extent possible with your brisk walk.
- Turn off your cell phone and other electronic devices about one hour before you go to bed.

Day Twenty-Four

Nutrition:

- Prepare your dinner tonight with my recovery superspices integrated into your dinner.
- While preparing and eating your meal and cleaning up, I recommend you practice my mindfulness meditations.
- Make sure to pack your midmorning and midafternoon snacks. If you need help with ideas, check out my list.
- Your carb cutoff should be around 5:00 p.m. this week.
- If you choose to have a late-night snack, choose from my list of recommended late-night snacks. If you are still craving carbs, have a teaspoon of MCT oil. That should calm down your brain.

Exercise:

- Keep your brisk walk in your routine today. If you are feeling up to it, extend the time frame to twenty to thirty minutes or beyond. If possible, walk in nature or a green setting. Also, feel free to do two brisk walks today. If you attempt two, bookend them at the beginning and end of your day to get the maximum benefit. If you plan to attend a twelve-step meeting, bookend both walks with your meeting, again to get the maximum benefit.
- If you are tracking your heart rate, keep your workouts in Zones 2 and 3 and, if you are comfortable doing so, challenge yourself to take it up to Zone 4 intermittently. However, go with what you feel is best for you, and make sure to keep your zone appropriate for your age, health, and ability.

Spirituality:

- Start your day with writing in your spiritual journal and integrating other morning self-care-based practices from our list of recommendations.
- After your morning self-care program, turn your cell phone and other electronic devices back on.
- Attend a twelve-step meeting and bookend it to the extent possible with your group activity.

Day Twenty-Five

Nutrition:

- Follow the same protocols that you did on day twenty-three by preparing breakfast and lunch today. Make sure to integrate my recovery superspices into both meals.
- Make sure to pack your midmorning and midafternoon snacks. If you need help with ideas, check out my list.
- Your carb cutoff should be around 5:00 p.m. this week.
- This evening, purchase and/or begin to prepare your dinners for later in the week. Make sure to integrate my mindfulness meditations while purchasing, preparing, and eating your meals all week.
- If you choose to have a late-night snack, choose from my list of recommended late-night snacks. If you are still craving carbs, have a teaspoon of MCT oil. That should calm down your brain.

Exercise:

- This morning include a group activity/workout of your choosing. If you cannot work out in the morning, then move this activity to late afternoon or early evening. Try to the extent possible to bookend this workout with your daily brisk walk.
- Make sure to take a brisk walk today of about fifteen to twenty minutes. If you are feeling up to it, extend the time to twenty to thirty minutes or beyond. If possible, walk in nature or a green setting. If you are feeling ambitious, add a second brisk walk into your day today.
- If you are tracking your heart rate, keep your workouts in Zones 2 and 3 and, if you are comfortable doing so, challenge yourself to

take it up to Zone 4 intermittently. However, go with what you feel is best for you, and make sure to keep your zone appropriate for your age, health, and ability.

Spirituality:
- Start your day by writing in your spiritual journal and integrating other morning self-care-based practices from my list of recommendations.
- Attend a twelve-step meeting and bookend it to the extent possible with your brisk walk.
- Shut off your cell phone and other electronic devices tonight about an hour before you go to bed.

Day Twenty-Six

Nutrition:
- Prepare your dinner tonight and include as many of my recovery superspices as you would like. While preparing and eating your meal and cleaning up, I recommend you practice our mindfulness meditations.
- Make sure to pack your midmorning and midafternoon snacks. If you need help with ideas, check out my list.
- Your carb cutoff should be around 5:00 p.m. this week.
- If you choose to have a late-night snack, choose from my list of recommended late-night snacks. If you are still craving carbs, have a teaspoon of MCT oil. That should calm down your brain.

Exercise:
- Keep a brisk walk in your routine today. If you are feeling up to it, extend the time frame to twenty to thirty minutes or beyond. If you can incorporate a second brisk walk of the same length, you will get the maximum benefit. If possible, bookend this and walk in nature or a green setting.
- If you are tracking your heart rate, keep your workouts in Zones 2 and 3 and, if you are comfortable doing so, challenge yourself to take it up to Zone 4 intermittently. However, go with what you feel is best for you, and make sure to keep your zone appropriate for your age, health, and ability.

Spirituality:

- Start your day by writing in your spiritual journal and integrating other morning self-care-based practices from my list of recommendations.
- After your morning self-care program, turn on your cell phone and other electronic devices.
- Attend a twelve-step meeting and bookend it to the extent possible with your group activity.

Day Twenty-Seven

Nutrition:

- Prepare your lunch for today and integrate my recovery superspices. While preparing and eating your meal and cleaning up, I recommend you practice my mindfulness meditations.
- Make sure to pack your midmorning and midafternoon snacks. If you need help with ideas, check out my list.
- Your carb cutoff should be around 5:00 p.m. this week.
- If you choose to have a late-night snack, choose from my list of recommended late-night snacks. If you are still craving carbs, have a teaspoon of MCT oil. That should calm down your brain.

Exercise:

- This morning include a group activity/workout of your choosing. If you cannot work out in the morning, then move this activity to late afternoon or early evening. Try to the extent possible to bookend this workout with your daily brisk walk.
- Keep your brisk walk in your routine today. If you are feeling up to it, extend the time frame to twenty to thirty minutes or beyond or add a second brisk walk at some point during the day. If possible, walk in nature or a green setting.
- If you are tracking your heart rate, keep your workouts in Zones 2 and 3 and, if you are comfortable doing so, challenge yourself to take it up to Zone 4 intermittently. However, go with what you feel is best for you, and make sure to keep your zone appropriate for your age, health, and ability.

Spirituality:
- Start your day by writing in your spiritual journal and integrating other morning self-care-based practices from my list of recommendations.
- Attend a twelve-step meeting and bookend it to the extent possible with your group activity.

Days Twenty-Eight and Twenty-Nine

My only recommendation for you is to celebrate one month of living clean, sober, and with self-care for body, mind, and spirit as your top priority. Here are my recommendations on how to celebrate. Take what works for you and leave the rest.

Nutrition:
- Prepare and then enjoy a home-cooked meal for your sponsor or someone in the program who is less fortunate.
- Work in as many healthy meals as you would like this weekend. If you decide to go outside of the Spiritual Adrenaline recommendations, try to incorporate as many nutritional tools as possible. For example, if you can cut off the carbs early and avoid late-night carb binges, that is progress.

Exercise:
- Attend yoga, Pilates, CrossFit, IntenSati, or another group activity that you enjoy.
- Attend a Y12SR meeting or yoga class.
- Go for a hike, bike ride, or jog in your local park.

Spirituality:
- Journal about how you feel after completing the seven-day detox and thirty-day Spiritual Adrenaline program.
- Journal about how you plan to continue to integrate outside issues into your recovery.
- Attend a twelve-step meeting and share about your experience.
- Review your journals from the past month and create a gratitude list.
- Send thank-you notes to anyone who inspired you to give this a try or who helped you during your journey.

Day Thirty

Today is about introspection and reflection. Your goal is to review your starting point, day one metrics, and spiritual journals, and make an assessment about where you are on day thirty. If you followed my seven-day detox and then implemented this program, this is day thirty-seven.

The biggest question is, How do you feel? Outward appearance is important, but how you feel on the inside is what matters most. How does your soul feel? For many, this may be the first time in your life that you paid so much attention to your health and needs. So how do you feel? Better, worse, or the same? What did you like most about the program? What did you like least?

Now's the time to inventory all three areas of the Spiritual Adrenaline program and assess what aspects you want to keep and those you don't, and maybe try other aspects for the first time. Make sure to inventory all three aspects of the Spiritual Adrenaline program: nutritional, exercise, and spiritual.

As you are about to transition to maintenance, it's important to put pen to paper and memorialize your experience, strength, and hope.

If you plan to continue with my maintenance program moving forward, use today to write in your spiritual journal about your aspirations for the next ninety days, six months, or more. What portions of your thirty-day plan do you want to continue, what do you want to change, and what are you are interested in trying to implement?

Think about whether to change your home group, keep your home group, check out new meetings, or integrate active fellowship into your program, and which of my spiritual tools you are interested in trying. Focus on whether the meetings you are attending work for you. Not all meetings work for everyone. The Twelve Steps are completely subjective. So the focus is not on whether certain meetings work for others—for example, if really hot people go to a certain meeting, or if there is some other external motivation to attend a specific meeting. You should be looking introspectively and asking whether the meeting or meetings you are attending work for you. Is the meeting the right one for you and helping to enrich your recovery? That is the only question that matters.

Spiritual Adrenaline Inspiration: Lisa Kreyling-Moore, Nevada

Lisa has been in recovery for twelve years. She abused alcohol and numerous drugs. Crystal meth became her favored drug of choice. In 2011, she founded Life Changes, Inc., a Reno, Nevada-based treatment program that specializes in treating women in recovery. This is what Lisa had to say about the importance of nutrition and exercise in recovery:

> I used meth for almost thirty years. I never liked the way I looked, and thought a size zero was healthy. Many years later, I realize how important nutrition truly is, and I am happy with my appearance.
>
> Exercise helps me cope with anxiety, stress, and cravings. Exercise, especially outdoors, allows me to breathe in fresh air and appreciate the beauty all around me. I take hikes and meditate and find huge stress relief.

Her message to newcomers is simple:

> Putting exercise and nutrition in your recovery is very important. We really do damage to ourselves while we are in active addiction. Once I got the healthy feeling that exercise gave me, I said I would never give this up. It became a healthy new addiction. Last, it's important that you find a higher power other than yourself to lean on.

CHAPTER FOURTEEN

Spiritual Adrenaline Maintenance

Now that you've completed your seven-day detox and your thirty-day plan, it's time for you to put together a four-week Spiritual Adrenaline Maintenance plan. After these four weeks, you are on your own to implement the tools in this book, those you learn about in the Spiritual Adrenaline online community, or some that you have created for yourself.

Keep these points in mind:

- Write in your spiritual journal about your goals for the next three months and beyond.
- Make sure to have your internal and external metrics tested and reviewed. If you need to update your prior metrics, please do so.
- Set reasonable and achievable nutrition, exercise, and spirituality goals.
- Think about how you can structure Spiritual Adrenaline around your family, work, business, and other commitments as you move forward.
- Confirm your twelve-step meetings and, to the extent possible, bookend them with exercise.

Maintenance: Month One
Nutritional Goals

Your nutritional goal this month is to prepare at least 25 percent of your meals at home throughout the week. If you are feeling ambitious, go for more. Hopefully, at this point you have reduced your caffeine intake to no more than two cups a day. You also should have been able to lower your sugar intake without sacrificing your sweet tooth.

I begin to introduce more of the Addiction Paleo program this month. First, I suggest you start to eat healthy fats in the morning along with protein and complex carbs. The majority of your meals should come from healthy fats and protein rather than carbs. You should be completely avoiding any processed carbs. I also suggest establishing a carb cutoff time between 3:00 and 5:00 p.m. A carb cutoff will help you lean out overnight as you sleep and make it harder to have carbs remaining to burn when you go to bed. The carb cutoff replaces having to count calories and macronutrients. If you need some carbs because you are getting irritable or otherwise are not feeling good after 7:00 p.m., go to my list of late-night snacks and choose items on that list from Chapter Eight.

Exercise Goals

This month, I suggest that you add in cardiovascular workouts in the Zone 3 range. You are up from Zone 1 and 2 workouts in the detox and four-week programs. However, "You do you," that is, go with what you feel is best for you and go at your own pace. Also, make sure you get your doctor's sign-off before beginning this or any other exercise program. For a refresher on the various zones, check out Chapter Ten. Keep challenging yourself and making your workouts progressively more challenging. Add some weight training to your schedule if you are feeling up to it. You should bookend your workouts with a meeting to maximize the benefits from both and to keep you in gratitude. Try to stick to the midday brisk walk, as this helps to break up long stretches at work or other commitments and gives you a break to refocus on self-care.

Spiritual Goals

After the seven-day detox and thirty-day program, you should have a pretty solid morning program, which should include journaling and/or reading recovery literature and/or meditation. During the thirty-day program you adjusted to turning off your electronic devices before going to bed and not turning them on until after your morning program. Aspire to three mornings a week, at the least, free of cell phone interruption. Again, I recommend turning off electronic devices at 9:00 p.m., but the actual time will vary based upon your life and personal or professional commitments.

Sunday

Sunday is a great day to pursue active fellowship, journal about your week, and purchase foods necessary for the week. All of these things are spiritual tools that will benefit you in ways you have yet to understand. Sundays are your days off. You can eat and do whatever you want; your only obligation for Sunday is to write a synopsis of your past week in your spiritual journal. Hopefully, you'll work some active fellowship into your ninety-day program on Sundays. But that's up to you.

Keep track of how your twelve-step and Spiritual Adrenaline programs affected you, what you liked, what you did not like, what kept you in gratitude, what irritated you or encouraged you to develop a resentment, or anything else that you feel is relevant.

For many of you, Sunday will be the day you check your external and internal measures. Use Sunday as a day for reflection and for getting you pumped up for the week ahead.

General Parameters

Overall, your daily lifestyle is becoming structured, which is necessary at this point and will pay off later, as the structure should help you form new nutrition, exercise, and spiritual habits in place of your old, unhealthy ones.

By now, you should look and feel very different from your day-one photo, blood work, and initial journal entries. You have demonstrated open-mindedness, honesty, and willingness, and you have embraced concepts that pushed you outside your recovery comfort zone.

Give yourself tremendous credit. Staying in your recovery comfort zone was easy. Challenging yourself to step out and integrate nutrition and exercise into your program while embracing new spiritual concepts can be difficult. Let's again look to the Twelve Steps for guidance. Have you practiced Steps Six and Seven and addressed character defects that may be undercutting your happiness and recovery? Step Ten asks you to continue to take personal inventory—including inventory of your physical, mental, and spiritual health—and when you were wrong, promptly admit it.

You've been journaling at least since we began the Spiritual Adrenaline program. Your journals record the food you eat, the amount and type of exercise you are doing, and your thoughts, feelings, and emotions on a daily basis.

Your emphasis on journaling and inventories is critical, as in active addiction many of us "never really acquired the habit of accurate self-appraisal. Working the Tenth Step becomes a regular part of everyday living, rather than unusual or set apart."[250] Spirituality and ritual are closely related; it's the ritual that can give an otherwise ordinary, everyday act spiritual meaning. Your journaling and inventories are necessary to avoid continuing resentments and damage to your body and mind, all of which "shut [you] off from the sunlight of the spirit."[251]

Put Your Metrics to Work
In Chapters Seven and Eight, you utilized various metrics to measure your internal and external health. Now is the time to review your metrics to ascertain what is working and what is not. If something isn't working, don't give up. Study the data you have accumulated over the past four months or so and evaluate what tweaks you can make to your Spiritual Adrenaline program to get the results you aspire to. Given that the program is totally customizable by you, maybe you will want to reevaluate if your goal was realistic or if a different goal or type of metric might be more appropriate for you as you keep moving forward in the right direction. For example, if you just started doing cardio and were hoping to lose two inches around your waist, that may not have happened. If you check your blood pressure, though, as a result of the cardio you might get a much healthier reading that in time will permit you to lose the inches.

The critical thing is to *never give up*. Once you throw in the towel, you lose. It's people who persevere who become the winners. They may get knocked down, but they always get back up.

Were Your Metrics Reasonable?

If you achieved your goals, you can skip this section. If you did not achieve your goals, this section is highly recommended. One of the most challenging things in recovery, and in anyone's life, is to become your own best friend rather than your own worst enemy. Both are learned behaviors, and you should strive toward the former rather than the later.

If you did not achieve the goal you set for yourself, think about whether or not it was reasonable given your health history, age, and life commitments such as family or a demanding job. If you just started to exercise for the first time in your life, realize that it takes time for the body to adjust and get in the rhythm of a new, active lifestyle. If you are over thirty, your metabolism isn't moving quite as fast as when you were twenty. This becomes even truer for people in their forties and fifties. The bottom line is that rather than giving up, reevaluate the goals you set for yourself, make necessary adjustments, and keep moving in a positive direction. Remember that it's progress, not perfection.

The first time you worked the steps was not something you could do on your own. You needed the guidance of a sponsor, someone who had been down the road before and could mentor you on how to do things smoothly. It wouldn't surprise me if many of you attempted to implement the Spiritual Adrenaline lifestyle without the guidance and support of a sponsor.

You need a twelve-step sponsor, but your Spiritual Adrenaline sponsor can be someone in recovery who has worked the steps, a personal trainer, a sports nutritionist, a registered dietician, or a trusted friend who can be honest with you. When you go it alone, it is almost always difficult to succeed. Beginners should not be expected to possess the skills of someone with exercise and nutrition experience under his or her belt. If you need a supportive community, check out the online community at www.spiritualadrenaline.com or my Facebook page. I suggest that you not hold yourself to the standard of an expert and then beat yourself up if you fail. That's the disease of addiction. Don't allow this to happen. Be your own best friend.

By asking for help and guidance you are not demonstrating weakness; you are demonstrating strength. You are keeping your ego in check and being honest with another human being about what you need. This is a spiritual practice. Don't be embarrassed or shy about asking for help or to admit you don't know everything. Trust me, nobody will criticize you for being honest, and you will improve very quickly with the proper guidance. How many times have you not put your hand up at a meeting when you wanted to share because you were shy or worried that people would think what you had to say was stupid? It's that "stinking thinking" again. If you had shared, it's likely that other people in the room would have related and gotten something out of it. They might even have come up to you and thanked you after the meeting.

Evaluate Your Blood Work with a Qualified Medical Professional

In Chapter Seven I recommended that everyone have their blood tested to ascertain the level of important markers. These markers tell the story of your overall health. Since you have a history of substance abuse, many of the important markers may not have been what you had hoped for. However, the body has an amazing capacity to heal, and after three or four months of living the Spiritual Adrenaline program and practicing its principles in all your affairs, your blood work should show some improvement.

Each of us has different genetics, a different health history, and a different addiction story, so your blood test results will be different from someone else's. Don't compare and despair, but rather go over your results with your doctor or another trusted medical professional. Here are some of the key markers and what you should look for:

White blood cell count: If you had a high white blood cell count, it may have been due to inflammation. After integration of healthy foods and exercise, your white blood cell count has hopefully been reduced. If it is not in the range you would like, keep going.

Glucose: Since a disproportionate number of people in recovery have either hypoglycemia or type 2 diabetes, if your blood work came back with high glucose levels, you are not alone. If you followed my nutritional recommendations, most importantly Addiction Paleo, your blood glucose level should be closer to the normal range. Remember that exercise also helps reduce blood glucose levels.

If you are not happy with your three-month or four-month measurement, don't give up; keep going and modify your program. Incorporate even healthier food choices and more exercise.

- **Cholesterol:** Has your HDL level increased? You should see some positive difference in your cholesterol levels if you have implemented my nutritional recommendations.
- **Cortisol:** Has your cortisol level increased or decreased? Discuss this with your doctor.
- **Triglycerides:** Has the level of triglycerides in your blood increased or decreased? You should see some positive difference if you implemented my nutritional recommendations.

Evaluate External Measures

Unlike your blood work that requires consultation with a trusted medical professional, your external measurements can be reviewed with your Spiritual Adrenaline sponsor, personal trainer, or sports nutritionist. Make sure it is someone who has also lived this program and/or has the professional certifications necessary to accurately assess your progress. Your journals now become critical so you can track your overall progress, try to assess what worked and what didn't, and then fine-tune your program moving forward to continue to see positive results. Let's go through a few of the major external measures.

- **Day One Photo:** If you took a photo on day one, take another one now. Make sure it is in the same place, with the same lighting, and first thing in the morning. Can you see a difference? Can your Spiritual Adrenaline sponsor, trainer, or other qualified person see differences that you cannot see? Aside from waist size or weight, do you see growth in your muscles? Does your skin look better? Does your hair look healthier? Really evaluate the contrasting photos for subtle changes. Change takes time; imagine your progress in six months to a year.
- **Weight:** If you chose this measurement, did you lose weight? Weight can be tricky because as you add muscle, your weight goes up. So if your goal was to add muscle and your weight went up, that is a positive thing. If your goal was to burn off fat reserves and lean out, it's probably not a positive thing. Whatever your goal was, use your

daily journal to figure out why your weight went up. If you practice rigorous honesty, you should be able to get to the bottom of why you did not achieve your goal and modify your Spiritual Adrenaline program accordingly.

- **Body Fat:** Unless you are an expert, it's difficult to determine body fat levels by eye. You need to have a way to measure. If you purchased a scale to measure, and it is the same scale you started with, you should be able to accurately track your body fat and ascertain whether you lost fat. If you succeeded in reducing your overall body fat, be proud. Excessive body fat puts stress on your ligaments, tendons, and joints; causes serious illnesses, including cardiovascular and liver disease; and negatively affects your self-esteem. If you did not achieve your goal, reformulate your strategy of applying Spiritual Adrenaline principles and keep going.

Spiritual Inventory
As you reflect on your journals, here are some suggested spiritual inventory questions to ponder:

- Are you the same person who started out on this journey?
- After living the principles of this program in all your affairs, has your level of fear dissipated?
- Has your anxiety been reduced?
- Has your overall stress level seemed more bearable?
- Do you sleep better?
- Have you begun a morning spiritual program?
- Does your morning program leave you feeling more positive throughout the day?
- Do you pay more attention at twelve-step meetings?
- Are you sharing more at meetings?
- Have you met more like-minded spiritual people who understand the importance of nutrition and exercise in their twelve-step program?
- Do you have more energy during the day?
- Are you less moody?
- Are you as reactive to impulses as you used to be?
- Do you take a deep breath before acting on an impulse?
- Have you been able to rein in your monkey mind?

- Are you managing your electronic devices rather than the devices managing you?
- Has your self-esteem improved?
- Is your recovery lifestyle more fun?
- Are you happier today than you were when you started this program?
- Aside from exercise and nutrition, what other outside issues are impacting your recovery, and how?

Keep journaling on how your life in recovery is evolving and becoming better. Continue to integrate Spiritual Adrenaline principles into all your affairs, and over time you will feel happier and healthier, with more consciousness of other people around you.

Spiritual Adrenaline Inspiration: **Sadie B., Oregon**

Sadie is in recovery from substance abuse. She says,

> Exercise and nutrition are self-love in action. I spent my whole life, including early recovery, stuffing myself numb with anything consumable—food, drugs, cigarettes, sex—whatever got the job done. Changing that behavior was imperative to getting well. My big shift came with yoga and running.
>
> From a young age I lacked the capacity to put space between my thoughts and my actions. Into adulthood, when the "thinking" brain is supposed to overcome the "emotional" brain, I was spontaneously combusting all over the place. Add a six-year meth addiction into the mix, and I was a recipe for disaster. In my first year of sobriety, *everything* was an emergency, especially my feelings. The meth had impacted my nervous system to such a degree that I couldn't sit still for five minutes, and my mind was always racing. I even inherited the nickname "Crisis." Running gave me a place to unpack all the excess energy I was lugging around. It cleared my mind and made me feel new again. Yoga took the years of pent-up rage and anxiety about past trauma and patiently unraveled it one breath at a time.

After a month of regular practice I realized I wasn't so quick to react; there was space between my thoughts and actions *for the first time ever*. The practices of yoga taught me to be slow, gentle, and kind to those around me and to myself, and that simple action brought my body, mind, and spirit into balance. Here's some advice:

- Pace yourself. Addicts fail because we demand instant gratification. Don't hit the pavement for the first time thinking you're going to run a 5K. Start with five minutes. Don't rearrange your whole diet. Make small changes one day at a time.
- Keep track of your progress. It's easy to forget where you were when you started. Having an "at-a-glance" record of how far you've come is important.
- Don't compare yourself to others. The only thing you need to surpass is your personal best. Stay committed and focused and you will succeed.

CHAPTER FIFTEEN

Dealing with Relapse

Relapse is a part of many people's stories. Relapse is by no means mandatory; however, it's also not the end of the world if you learn and grow from the experience. I always admire folks at meetings who raise their hands after a relapse and start their day count all over again. That's a surefire way to kick your addiction's ass and take away its power over you.

Raising your hand and starting over takes tremendous courage. Often, people are too ashamed to admit their relapse. (I include myself in this group my first time around.) Being ashamed is a problem since hesitation in acknowledging a mistake runs counter to the rigorous honestly suggested by the Twelve Steps. In the not-too-distant future, there will likely be some innovative technologies to help lessen the chances of relapse. For example, in 2016, Italian researchers published the results of a study that measured the success of electrical stimulation of the prefrontal cortex in cocaine addicts. The prefrontal cortex is the part of the brain responsible for our ability to reason and use judgment, critical to breaking the cycle of relapse. In people using stimulants like cocaine, this part of the brain is typically underutilized. The reason? Drug-damaged neural pathways. Researchers are using electrical charges to the prefrontal cortex in much the same manner as a reboot on a frozen computer.

Twenty-nine cocaine addicts interested in quitting were recruited for the study. Sixteen underwent one month of daily brain stimulation while thirteen received standard care, including medication for anxiety and depression. By the end of the trial, eleven people in the brain-stimulation-only group were drug-free, while only three in the other group remained that way.[252] One of the participants stated that after the first electrical stimulation session he "felt calm." He stopped using and has remained abstinent. When asked to describe how this type of treatment helped, the participant said, "It was a complete change," and described a "feeling of vitality and desire to live, which [he] had not felt for a long This rapidly progressing world with its ever-increasing faster tempo of living demands that we be physically fit and alert in order that we may succeed in the unceasing race with keen competition, which rewards the 'go-getter' but bypasses the 'no-getter. time." Large-scale studies on this technology are presently underway.

It is true that this technology might be able to help some of you in the very near future. But other ways to stimulate your prefrontal cortex are available to you *right here and now*. MRIs of the brains of people who engage in cardiovascular exercise, yoga, and mediation have confirmed that these activities stimulate the prefrontal cortex. In fact, the longer you continue exercising, the better results you see in the context of improved brain function. Moreover, a 2015 study is among the few to study the molecular neurobiology of twelve-step programs.[253] Although only preliminary findings have been released, early results demonstrate some improvement in prefrontal cortex activity as a result of step work and participation in a twelve-step fellowship.[254]

So while you look forward to any technologies that can lessen your chances of relapse, so much of what |the Spiritual Adrenaline program recommends will help stimulate your brain in the right places to reduce your chances of relapse *right now*. The solution is here if you choose to avail yourself of it.

With that said, here are some additional recommended relapse-prevention tools.

People, Places, and Things

I used to hate it when people would mention the need to change people, places, and things. My first go-around, I wanted to continue to hang out in bars with the same friends who were drinking and using drugs, and basically to live the same lifestyle I had lived as a practicing alcoholic and addict as a "sober" person. Today I realize that I was not sober back then, but rather dry or abstinent. Truly sober people who are embracing the principles of recovery do not want to hang out with active alcoholics and addicts in the same miserable dark places that ruined their lives while they were in active addiction.

There is no doubt about it; people, places, and things make all the difference in the world. To succeed in recovery and find happiness, you've got to do your inventories and take the necessary actions to change the people, places, and things that are interrelated with your alcohol and other drug use.

The Spiritual Adrenaline lifestyle helps prevent relapse since people, places, and things in your life will naturally change as a consequence of step work and action. For example, by joining a gym and taking a small group-fitness class, you will be in a new place around a new group of people—very different from the days of your active using—and doing a new activity. The benefits of the Spiritual Adrenaline program will result as a natural consequence of right action.

When you live the Spiritual Adrenaline lifestyle, you are creating layers of protection that separate you from your substance of choice. Think of your recovery as living in a castle surrounded by three moats: the first moat is nutrition, the second is exercise, and the third is spirituality. The healthy habits you've established over the last few weeks should make it less likely that you'll act out on impulse, a precursor to relapse. For example, if you are not ingesting lots of sugar and caffeine, you avoid getting hyper, having major mood swings, and being unable to resist impulsive thinking. You've developed healthy coping tools, including exercise and meditation, that enable you to handle stressors in a way that benefits your recovery. For instance, when you're irritated with somebody or something, go to the gym, do yoga, or take a hike in order to work it through rather than hanging out at a bar or visiting your drug dealer. Your spiritual practice, including morning meditation and reading from your journals, will keep you in gratitude even when you find the day challenging.

Common Early Warning Signs

There are a number of well-recognized early warning signs that you are at risk for a relapse. Just because you experience one or more of these does not mean a relapse is imminent. It may just mean that you are dealing with a major issue in your life and you need a break from your normal routine. You know yourself better than anyone else. Trust your instincts and practice rigorous honesty with yourself.

Here's a list of common relapse warning signs:

- You feel a loss of gratitude.
- You stop attending meetings.
- You stop sharing at meetings.
- You lose interest in step work and journaling.
- You stop going to the gym or exercising.
- You stop eating in a healthy way.
- You stop speaking to your sponsor.
- You feel a general attitude of "fuck it."
- You act out sexually or financially (for example, go on shopping binges) or exhibit other compulsive behaviors.
- You refuse to deal with critical medical issues.
- You refuse to deal with critical financial issues such as paying taxes.
- You glamorize your using friends and using days.
- You hang out around bars or other places associated with your past using.
- You do not get adequate sleep.
- You get defensive when confronted about changes in your behavior.
- You experience the inability to work through common emotions.

If you begin to experience these factors, my best advice is to do the opposite of what that little voice in your head, that is, your addiction, is telling you. If the voice is telling you not to go to a meeting, go to two meetings that day if you can. If it is telling you not to go to the gym, go to the gym. Try to do the opposite, and if you can, reach out to someone in your support network who has been there and can relate.

Burning Desire

The strong desire to use is commonly referred to in twelve-step meetings as a burning desire. Many meetings set aside time for people with a burning desire to share. If you have a burning desire, get yourself to a meeting, and if you need to share right away, don't hesitate to get your hand up and let people know. Others will understand, as they have been there and will listen and likely offer advice and fellowship. Whatever tool you choose to utilize, don't be ashamed to ask for help. It is a sign of strength rather than weakness; asking for help confirms that your disease is no longer in control of your thoughts and actions. This is part of becoming emancipated from the mental slavery of addiction.

Your 911 List

A very helpful tool when you are feeling overwhelmed by the impulse to use is a 911 list, either on your electronic devices or printed out and hanging someplace at home. I came up with this tool based upon my own experience with relapse my first time in recovery. I realized that when I would relapse, I would get an impulsive thought, act on it, and have had a drink or snorted a line by the time I actually realized what was happening. I basically remembered nothing between the impulse and the using, and by the time I realized what was happening, it was too late.

My 911 list includes effective tools that I knew worked for me. I created a top-ten list of these tools and put it right on my phone and iPad. My list includes calling my sponsor (who is a certified sports nutritionist and personal trainer); listening to music with a positive message; reading my old journals from rehab and my first couple of years of recovery; hydrating with water; going to the gym and working out, swimming, or doing yoga or Pilates; going to church; deep breathing; getting out into nature; and going to a meeting. When I would get an impulse, I would hit my 911 list and suddenly the tools that worked for me popped up. It became a habit early on; as soon as I would feel an impulse, I would stop what I was doing and go right to my 911 list. As each of us is different, what works for me and what might work for you are not the same thing, but by creating your own personalized 911 list, you can shut down impulsive thinking by recovery-oriented guidance from a tool that works for you.

Relapse Inventory

If you experienced a relapse, remember that it's not the end of the world. I've been there and I am here to tell you that you can come back stronger than ever if you look at relapse as an opportunity to learn and grow. Pick yourself back up and get right back into your recovery. Journal about the experience and inventory the causes, the experiences, and what you learned as a result.

You might want to review your inventory with your sponsor or someone you trust in the program to talk through the issues and get honest feedback. Here's my inventory in the form of a questionnaire:

1. What person, place, and/or thing triggered my relapse?
2. In what way did each trigger me to use?
3. How did I put myself in a position where it was easy to use?
4. Was I hungry, angry, lonely, or tired when I relapsed? If so, why and how can I avoid that in the future?
5. To avoid another relapse, what people, places, and things do I need to avoid?
6. What did I learn from my relapse?
7. What people do I need to avoid in the future? What people are positive and support my recovery?
8. What places do I need to avoid in the future? What places are positive and support my recovery?
9. What things do I need to avoid in the future? What things are positive and support my recovery?
10. What steps can I take next time when the urge to use arises?

Relapse Action Plan

After you complete your relapse inventory, it's time to develop an action plan. Nothing happens in the Twelve Steps by accident; you have to do the work. The work is based upon taking action. Your life is too important to not go about future relapse prevention without an effective plan. Obviously, everyone's action plan will be different based upon his or her personal circumstances and experience. You should run your action plan by your sponsor or other trusted person to get feedback on whether your proposed plan is reasonable, has adequate self-care-based amends that will benefit you, and is not unrealistic or otherwise unachievable.

The Importance of Gratitude

This is from AA's *Daily Reflections:* "When beaming with gratitude, one's heartbeat must surely result in outgoing love." Probably the most potent antirelapse tool available to anyone in addiction recovery is gratitude. There's a saying in the twelve-step world: "A grateful alcoholic or addict will not drink or use."

In a 2016 study, researchers tracked sixty-seven individuals following inpatient treatment. Among the conclusions of the study is this: "If a client does not want to change or is ambivalent about change, a gratitude practice might affirm what is good in life while currently drinking. However, if a client has made a decision to change and has thereby entered the action stage, then a gratitude practice should affirm changes already underway."[255]

One sure way to stay in gratitude is to read journals from when you were just starting out in recovery. When you write things down in your journal, changes get memorialized, as do the tools you have used in the past to overcome challenges. When you go back and read past journals, it reinforces that over time and with hard work, you can change and grow in a positive way. It's too easy to forget positive progress you have made. You wind up being your own worst critic, which makes it easier to engage in self-defeating behaviors. Remember the "critical parent"?

Your journals are a window into your soul. It's your story of personal growth as a result of the hard work you have put into your program. By seeing your growth reflected in black-and-white and in your own words, it makes it much less likely you will use going forward.

Spiritual Adrenaline Inspiration: Sean S., New York

Sean S. is cofounder of ROCovery Fitness in Rochester, New York. He is a recovering alcoholic. Sean was an athlete in high school, joined the military after graduating, and wanted to become an Army Ranger. In his formative years and in the years after joining the military, Sean would go from hard-core physical training to binge drinking that would last for days. For medical reasons, which he later found out were related to his drinking, Sean was unable to join the Rangers. He served his country as a member of the infantry in Afghanistan. During his first tour of duty, he trained and fought, dried out, and served with valor.

Upon returning from Afghanistan, he resumed his hard-core binge drinking. He ultimately suffered an alcohol withdrawal seizure. Over the next three years, he was in and out of three inpatient and four outpatient substance abuse treatment facilities. He describes himself as a chronic relapser who "relied on exercise and pure will to stay sober." He returned overseas to Kuwait for a second deployment. During this time he stayed focused and sober, only to relapse again three months after returning home.

After relapsing, Sean was, as he describes himself, a "drunk who was jobless and homeless." He was sent to a veterans' halfway house. Along with the other "misfit vets" there, he developed a routine centered on exercise, working out, and meetings. Sean's National Guard unit stood by him. The light bulb finally went on in his head. After being clean for a period of time, he was offered the opportunity to go to the U.S. Army Ranger School and completed the training and eventually competed in the Best Ranger competition. He went back to school and received a degree in addiction counseling. He describes his life then as "having a program of recovery as well as a healthy lifestyle centered on health, wellness, fitness, and nutrition that truly complement each other."

CHAPTER SIXTEEN

Living Beyond Your Self-Imposed Limitations

Like the Twelve Steps, the Spiritual Adrenaline program is a design for living. It's not something to be followed for a short while like a fad diet, and then abandoned once you achieve your goals. It's a lifelong commitment to a healthy way of life, taken one day at a time. Nowhere in twelve-step literature does it state that the steps are to be worked once and then abandoned. In fact, the steps are designed to be continuously worked and integrated into your daily life, habits, and lifestyle.

If you practice the twelve-step principles in all your affairs, you won't need to sit down and actually "work" the steps, as you will be living your step work and reaping the rewards. In fact, the more you integrate step work into your daily plan for living, the more you will grow, and your goals and aspirations will continue to grow as well. That's the beauty of this way of life.

In *Just for Today,* self-imposed limitations are described as follows:

Most of us come to the program with a multitude of self-imposed limitations that kept us from realizing our full potential, limitations that impede our attempts to find the value that lie at the core of our being. We place limitations on our ability to be true to ourselves, limitations on our ability

257

to function at work, limitations on the risks we're willing to take—the list seems endless.[256]

Like me, hopefully one day you will come to believe that along with your higher power, you are capable of anything—even moving mountains. If you cannot move them, you can climb them for sure!

When you see your blood work come back with a substantial reduction in your blood sugar; when you see how cravings can be reduced by reducing your sugar, junk food, and caffeine intake; when you see inches disappear from around your waist; when you see the twinkle come back into your eye; when you begin to feel positive energy emanate from the deepest part of your soul; when you begin to hear compliments from others about how your actions and appearance have changed for the better; and when your loved ones share with you how proud they are of you for the changes you have made in your life, health, and new recovery—the changes you have chosen to make become hardwired in you. Now that you realize you cannot succeed in isolation, but rather that you are interrelated with those in the world around you, then you will want to share your positive energy with others one day at a time.

The key to the steps is to integrate them into your daily life, and, as you grow and change, how you apply the steps to your personal circumstances will change as well. For example, I was not in good health in the fall of 2011 and near bankruptcy when I first worked the steps. Now, almost eight years later, I am healthy and financially secure. However, I have a whole different set of challenges facing me. The steps continue to empower me to address those issues. Just like the day will never come when I stop going to the gym because I have achieved all of my fitness goals, I will never stop working the steps because I have been "cured." It's a lifelong commitment that changes as we change and that we take one day at a time, one rep at a time, one meal at a time, and one breath at a time.

I hope that after reading *Spiritual Adrenaline,* you no longer fear change. No one likes change, least of all alcoholics and addicts, but life really amounts to a series of changes, one after the other.

The present moment only lasts for a second; then that moment becomes the past and there is no guarantee that anything will remain the same. The Buddhist concept of impermanence has helped me, and millions of others, recognize that change will happen regardless of our attempts to cling to the past.

It's true that we must learn to let go lest we be dragged. By practicing the Twelve Steps and integrating the Spiritual Adrenaline lifestyle into your practice, it becomes easier to let go of the past and embrace rather than fear change, as the changes in our lives are increasingly positive.

Sure, we all have to deal with the difficult things that life throws our way: death, disease, depression, taxes, and bad relationships, to name a few. But with our minds, bodies, and spirits healthy, and with effective tools at our disposal, these challenges can be embraced rather than feared. From the new heights you may achieve, you can look down on your past addiction as a gift that was necessary to teach you the art of living. Rather than being embarrassed or feeling guilty, you may embrace it and continue to grow.

I never thought I would be where I am today when I finally made the decision to stop torturing my body and soul and embrace recovery on May 11, 2011. I just wanted to be restored to physical health and sanity. I wanted my loved ones to have peace and not be constantly worried about what will happen next.

My mother is eighty-nine years old. When the day inevitably comes when she passes on, I do not want her last thoughts to be filled with worry and anxiety about me. Rather than anxious and worried, I want her to be at peace. I want her to be able to reflect on how beautiful her life has been and all the joy our family has shared, those beautiful memories that will truly last forever. I want her to pass with the knowledge that I will be healthy and happy. This is the simple joy that Spiritual Adrenaline has made possible for me and my family. For me, material things mean very little. Rather, what matters are things that cannot be given a price tag. Serenity, for me and my loved ones, is the most valuable gift I have been given. It's a simple gift that I can keep only by sharing it with others.

This passage from *Drop the Rock* sums it up: "To become the person we can be, we must drop the rock [to end] all the grasping and holding on to old practices of behaving and thinking that are harmful to ourselves and others." If your twelve-step lifestyle is getting stale, making you live in a small comfort zone that seems to grow smaller all the time, a sincere attempt to work the steps while living the Spiritual Adrenaline lifestyle is a good choice. It can take you to new places and a life well beyond your self-imposed limitations.

This is serenity and true emotional sobriety and recovery achieved by practicing the principles of the Twelve Steps in all your affairs.

Resources

Spiritual Adrenaline Online Community
www.spiritualadrenaline.com

Facebook: @SpiritualAdrenaline
Instagram: spiritual_adr
Twitter: @spiritualadren
Email: tom@spiritualadrenaline.com

Books
Highly Recommended

Drop the Rock: Removing Character Defects—Steps Six and Seven, Bill P., Todd W., Sara S., Hazelden Foundation Publishing (1993)

Drop the Rock . . . The Ripple Effect: Using Step 10 to Work Steps 6 and 7 Every Day, Fred H., Hazelden Foundation Press (2016)

Cracking the Metabolic Code: 9 Keys to Optimal Health, James LaValle, Basic Health Publications (2004)

Fitness

Eat to Be Fit, Michael J. Foley and Pat Walsh, Living Well Publishing Company (2002)

The IntenSati Method, Patricia Moreno, Simon Spotlight Entertainment (2009)

Return to Life Through Contrology, Joseph H. Pilates and William John Miller, Presentation Dynamics (2012). Originally published in 1945.

Recovery 2.0, Tommy Rosen, Hay House (2014)

Sugar and Recovery

Simply Sugar Free, Sue Brown, Promoting Natural Health, LLC (2014)

The Sugar Smart Diet, Anne Alexander, Rodale Publishing (2013)

Junk Foods & Junk Moods, Lindsey Smith, www.foodmoodgirl.com (2012)

Sugar Detox for Beginners, Josh West, Hayward Press (2013)

Sweet Nothings: Safe or Scary? The Inside Scoop on Sugar Substitutes, Nutrition Action, Annual Report (2014)

General Nutrition

A New View of Healthy Eating, Melanie A. Albert, Experience Nutrition Group, LLC (2016)

Caveman Doctor, www.cavemandoctor.com

General Nutrition and Recovery

Seven Weeks to Sobriety, Dr. John Mathews Larson, First Ballantine Books (1997)

Under the Influence, Dr. James R. Milam and Katherine Ketcham, Bantam Books (1983)

Nutritional Supplements, Joe Canon, MS, Infinity Publishing (2008)

Eating Right to Live Sober, Katherine Ketcham and Dr. L. Ann Mueller, Writers House Publishing (1986)

Food for Recovery, Dr. Joseph D. Beasley and Susan Knightly, Crown Publishing (1993)

The Vitamin Cure for Alcoholism, Dr. Abram Hoffer and Dr. Andrew W. Saul, Basic Health Publications (2008)

Depression Free Naturally, Dr. Joan Matthews Larson, Random House (2001)

Potatoes Not Prozac, Kathleen DesMaisons, PhD, Simon & Schuster (1998)

Water: You're Not Sick, You're Thirsty, F. Batmanghelidj, Global Health Solutions, Inc. (2008)

Caffeinated, Murray Carpenter, Hudson Street Press (2014)

Buddhism and Recovery

The Twelve Step Buddhist, Darren Littlejohn, Simon & Schuster (2009)

Refuge Recovery, Noah Levine, HarperCollins (2014)

Against the Stream, Noah Levine, Harper One (2007)

Interconnected, Ogyen T. D. Karmapa, Wisdom Publications (2017)

The Heart Is Noble, Ogyen T. D. Karmapa, Wisdom Publications (2012)

Ordinary Recovery, William Alexander, Shambhala (2014)

1325 Buddhist Ways to Be Happy, Barbara Ann Kipfer, Ulysses Press (2007)

Yoga and Recovery

The Yoga Sutras of Patanjali, Fourth Edition, Translation and Commentary by Sri Swami Satchidananda, Integral Yoga Publications (2015)

Yoga and the Twelve-Step Path, Kyczy Hawk, Central Recovery Press (2012)

Yogic Tools for Recovery, Kyczy Hawk, Central Recovery Press (2017)

The Yogic Tools Workbook, Kyczy Hawk, Central Recovery Press (2018)

The Twelve Steps and Christian Faith

The Life Recovery Bible, Second Edition, New Living Translation (2013)

Daily Meditation and Reflection

The Language of Letting Go, Melody Beattie, Hazelden Foundation (1990)

Daily Reflections, Alcoholics Anonymous World Services (2011)

Just for Today, Narcotics Anonymous World Services (2009)

The Power of Now, Eckhart Tolle, Namaste Publishing (1997)

Meditation
Meditation for Beginners, Jack Kornfield, Sounds True, Inc. (2008)

General Recovery
Alcoholics Anonymous, Fourth Edition, Alcoholics Anonymous World Services (2001)

Living Sober, Alcoholics Anonymous World Services, Inc. (1998)

Back to Basics, Wally P., Faith with Works Publishing (1997)

Your Blood Never Lies, James LaValle, Square One Publishers (2013)

Impact of Prescription Medication on Nutrient Retention
Drug Muggers, Suzy Cohen, Rodale Publishers (2011)

LGBT (Recovery)
Coming Out Spiritually, Christian de la Huerta, Penguin (1999)

Smoking Cessation
Allen Carr's Easy Way to Stop Smoking, Allen Carr's Easyway International (2011)

Nicotine Anonymous, Fourth Edition, Nicotine Anonymous World Services (2008)

General
The Tools, Phil Stutz and Barry Michels, Spiegel & Grau (2012)

General Information
Medical

Dr. Michael Bedecs
Age Management Center
www.agemanagementcenter.com
Portland, ME (207) 747-1435
Jupiter, FL (561) 331-6483

Nutrition Counseling

Mike Foley
Foley Fitness
Facebook: @mikefoleyfitness
www.mikefoleyfitness.com
mfoley2000@hotmail.com

Organizations

Addict2Athlete
Stay Invincible CrossFit
2101 East Evans
Pueblo, CO 81004
Facebook: @WeareSICrossFit
www.addict2athlete.org
rob@addict2athlete.org
(719) 250-7805

ROCovery Fitness
1035 Dewey Avenue
Rochester, NY 14613
www.ROCoveryfitness.org
mail@rocoveryfitness.org
(585) 484-0234

The Phoenix
2233 Champa Street
Denver, CO 80205
www.thephoenix.org
mail@thephoenix.org
(720) 440-9175

Temperance Training
Boca Raton, FL
temperancetraining.org
Facebook: @Temperance Training
info@temperancetraining.org
(925) 705-5340

Yoga of Twelve Step Recovery (Y12SR)
www.y12sr.com

Rise & Grind Reno
Facebook: @riseandgrindreno
Grant Denton: Facebook: @grant denton

Life Changes Reno
Lisa Kreyling: lisa@lifechangesinc.org
www.lifechanges.org
(773) 685-8145

The IntenSati Method
www.intensati.com

Recovery 2.0
www.recovery2point0.com

Refuge Recovery
www.refugerecovery.org

Yoga of Recovery
www.yogaofrecovery.com

Smoking Cessation
_____

Allen Carr's Easy Way to Stop Smoking
www.allencarr.online
www.theeasywaytostopsmoking.com

Spiritual Adrenaline Inspirations Contact Information
Preface

Kallup McCoy II
RezHope
Cherokee, NC
Facebook: @Kallup McCoy II; @rezhope
mccoykallup@icloud.com

Chapter One

Scott Richardson
Normal, IL
Facebook: @scottrichardsonBN

Chapter Two

Yana Khasphar
ROCovery Fitness
Rochester, NY
www.rocoveryfitness.org
Instagram: @rocoveryfitness
yana@rocoveryfitness.org

Chapter Three

Nancy C.
Nancy has asked that her contact information remain anonymous.

Chapter Four

Willa Wirth
Portland, ME
Facebook: @WillaWirth

Chapter Five

Sheena Archuleta
Pueblo, CO
www.addict2athlete.org
Instagram: @addict2athlete
sheena@addict2athlete.org

Chapter Six

Holly Faurot
New York, NY
Facebook: @Holly Faurot
holly.faurot@gmail.com

Chapter Seven

Tim Mustion
Boca Raton, FL
Facebook: @TemperanceTraining; @timmy_musti
Instagram: @temperancetraining
temperancetraining@gmail.com

Chapter Eight

Alex Ferrer
Cabarete, Dominican Republic
Facebook: @alexferrer
Ferrerfitness@icloud.com

Chapter Nine

Austin C.
Austin has asked that his contact information remain anonymous.

Chapter Ten

Clayton Young
Houston, Texas
Twitter: @Fit2Four7
Instagram: @c.y.2.lift
Evolveclay22@gmail.com

Chapter Eleven

Kyczy Hawk
San Jose, CA
www.yogarecovery.com
kyczy@yogarecovery.com

Chapter Twelve
Rob Archuleta
Pueblo, CO
www.addict2athlete.org
Instagram: @addict2athlete
rob@addict2athlete.org

Chapter Thirteen
Lisa Kreyling-Moore
Reno, NV
www.lifechangesinc.org
lisa@lifechangesinc.org
(775) 685-8145

Chapter Fourteen
Sadie Barr
Grants Pass, OR
www.sadiebarryoga.com
Facebook: @sadie barr yoga
sadiejbarr@gmail.com

Chapter Fifteen
Sean Smith
ROCovery Fitness
Rochester, NY
sean@rocoveryfitness.org
Instagram: @rocoveryfitness

Spiritual Adrenaline Recipes

Breakfast Recipes

All of these recipes should be supplemented with green vegetables, for example, kale, spinach, broccoli, watercress, or asparagus. I also recommend adding in half an avocado or organic peanut or almond butter to provide your body with fat for energy. If you would like bread, Ezekiel bread is a great choice along with whole wheat or multigrain. If you like bacon, it's okay to work in turkey-bacon once or twice a week.

STEEL CUT OATMEAL WITH CINNAMON, BLUEBERRIES, AND HONEY

INGREDIENTS:

- 1 cup steel-cut oatmeal (This means *not* the quick cooking or instant version.)
- 4 cups water
- 1 tsp. cinnamon (You can substitute nutmeg or other recovery superspices.)
- ½ cup blueberries (You can substitute strawberries, bananas, blackberries, or your other favorites.)
- Honey or other sweetener to your preference

Preparation: Heat water to boil. Once boiling, add oats, cinnamon, and blueberries. Reduce heat to low or medium and cover. Cook for about fifteen minutes or until ready. Stir frequently.

Preparation time: Fifteen to twenty minutes.

Additional substitutions: Organic peanut or almond butter, walnuts, almonds, or other nuts or seeds.

Sweet Potato Pancakes

INGREDIENTS:

- 1 sweet potato
- 2 eggs
- Cinnamon to preference
- Fruit to preference

Preparation: Heat oven to 325 F. Remove the skin from the sweet potato and roast until softens (to save time, microwave and then roast). Put softened sweet potato in blender and mix with two eggs and spices of your choosing. Mix well. Heat a griddle or frying pan over medium heat. Lightly oil with coconut or olive oil. Pour batter onto heated griddle or frying pan and cook for five to seven minutes. Use two spatulas to turn pancake over. Once turned, allow to cook another three to five minutes.

Preparation time: Thirty minutes.

Additional substitutions: Organic peanut butter, walnuts, almonds, or other nuts or seeds, any of my recovery superspices, fruit such as blueberries.

Everything Veggie Omelet

INGREDIENTS:

- 2 or 3 eggs
- Any of superfood veggies (the more color the better)
- Coconut oil

Preparation: Grease frying pan with coconut oil. Break eggs into bowl, beat eggs, and stir in vegetables. The more color the better. Cook on medium heat until egg firms, turning when necessary.

Preparation time: Time varies.

Milk and Honey Chilled Overnight Chia

INGREDIENTS:

- 2 cups steel cut oats
- 4 tbsp. chia seeds
- 4 tbsp. honey
- Almond or coconut milk

Preparation: In a twelve- to sixteen-ounce jar, add oats, chia seeds, honey, and milk. Cover and shake well or mix in blender. Refrigerate overnight. Enjoy the next day.

Preparation time: Ten minutes.

Blueberry or Banana Chilled Overnight Flax

INGREDIENTS:

- 2 cups steel cut oats
- 4 tbsp. flax seeds
- 4 tbsp. honey
- 1 cup blueberries or 1 banana
- Almond or coconut milk

Preparation: In a twelve- to sixteen-ounce jar, add oats, chia seeds, honey, and milk. Cover and shake well or mix in blender. Refrigerate overnight.

Preparation time: Ten minutes.

Lunch Recipes

All of these recipes should be supplemented with green vegetables, for example, kale, spinach, broccoli, watercress, or asparagus. I also recommend adding a healthy fat and, if you would like bread, Ezekiel bread is a great choice along with whole wheat or multigrain. Make sure to work in at least one leafy green and some recovery superspices.

CHICKEN, TURKEY BACON, AND AVOCADO SALAD

INGREDIENTS:

- 1 6 to 8 oz. chicken breast
- 1 ripe avocado
- ½ cup turkey bacon
- Veggies of your choosing
- Watercress and mesclun salad (mix evenly)
- Extra virgin olive oil

Preparation: Grill chicken breast until golden brown and to your preference. Chop avocado and then mix with turkey bacon. Add veggies of your choosing from my recovery superfoods in Chapter Nine. Mix over watercress or mesclun salad and add olive oil or other dressing of your choice.

Preparation time: Twenty minutes.

CHICKEN OR SALMON WALNUT, STRAWBERRY, AND PISTACHIO SALAD

INGREDIENTS:

- Chicken breast (6 oz.) or salmon (8 oz.)
- ½ cup walnuts
- 1 cup strawberries
- ½ cup pistachios
- Watercress and mesclun salad (mix evenly)
- Extra virgin olive oil

Preparation: Grill chicken breast or salmon in coconut oil; mix walnuts, strawberries, and pistachios in a baking bowl. Grill chicken breast or salmon until golden brown and to your preference. Add veggies of your choosing from my recovery superfoods in Chapter Nine. Mix over watercress and mesclun salad and add olive oil or other dressing of your choice.

Preparation time: Twenty minutes.

Turkey, Chicken, Salmon, or Veggie Sandwich with Half Bun

INGREDIENTS:

- Your choice of fish, turkey, or veggies
- Your choice of fixings, such as lettuce, tomato, onion, pickles, etc.
- ½ of a whole wheat or multigrain bun or role
- Spicy mustard, mayo, veggie ketchup
- Recovery superspices

Preparation: Create your own super sandwich from any of the ingredients included above. Mix with healthy fixings, recovery superspices, and healthy condiments. If you would like, add goat cheese or another cheese as a treat.

Preparation time: Ten minutes.

Dinner Recipes

All of these recipes should be supplemented with green vegetables, for example, kale, spinach, broccoli, watercress, or asparagus.

Oven Roasted Chicken Breasts with Superspices

INGREDIENTS:

- 4 free-range, antibiotic-free chicken breasts (4–6 oz. each)
- 2 tsp extra-virgin olive oil.
- 4 tsp recovery superspices of your choosing
- Pinch of black pepper
- Pinch of sea salt

Preparation: Preheat oven to 375. Lay chicken breasts into baking dish. Sprinkle superspices, black pepper, and sea salt on the top of breasts. Place in oven and bake until golden brown or to your liking.

Preparation time: Fifteen to twenty minutes.

GRASS-FED BEEF BURGER

INGREDIENTS:

- 1 lb. grass-fed beef (makes about four 6 oz. burgers)
- Half whole wheat bun
- One tomato
- One onion
- Romaine lettuce
- 2 tsp. extra-virgin olive oil
- 4 tsp. recovery superspices of your choosing
- Pinch of black pepper
- Pinch of sea salt

Preparation: Mix grass-fed ground beef with olive oil, superspices of your choosing, black pepper, and sea salt. Make sure all ingredients are evenly distributed in the beef. Chop onions, tomatoes, and other toppings. Grill on oven using medium heat for about seven to fifteen minutes or when done to your preference.

Preparation time: Twenty minutes.

BAKED SALMON

INGREDIENTS:

- 4 wild salmon fillets (6 to 8 oz. each) Avoid farm-raised salmon.
- ½ tbsp. extra virgin olive oil
- 4 tsp. recovery superspices of your choosing
- Pinch of black pepper
- Pinch of sea salt

Preparation: Preheat oven to 325. Lay wild salmon into baking dish. Sprinkle superspices, black pepper, and sea salt onto the top of the fish. Place in oven and bake until golden brown or to your liking.

Preparation time: Fifteen to twenty minutes.

BAKED SEA BASS WITH TOMATO, PARSLEY, ONION, AND SUPERSPICES

INGREDIENTS:

- 4 sea bass filets (6 to 8 oz. each)
- 1 tomato
- 1 onion
- 4 parsley sprigs
- ½ tbsp. extra-virgin olive oil
- 4 tsp. recovery superspices of your choosing
- Pinch of black pepper
- Pinch of sea salt

Preparation: Preheat oven to 325. Lay sea bass into baking dish. Sprinkle extra-virgin olive oil, superspices, black pepper, sea salt, and parsley onto the top of the fish. Dice tomato and onions and sprinkle over the fish. Place in oven and bake until golden brown or to your liking.

Preparation time: Fifteen to twenty minutes.

TURKEY TACOS

INGREDIENTS:

- 1 lb. ground turkey meat
- Taco shells (gluten free)
- Taco seasoning or your own seasoning with recovery superspices
- 1 tomato
- 1 onion
- Shredded cheese (either your own or in the package)
- ¼ cup water
- Hot sauce (to your preference)

Preparation: Cook ground turkey meat at medium heat on oven and stir frequently to make sure all the meat cooks. As the turkey meat browns and is almost done, mix in your pre-purchased taco seasoning mix or create your own using recovery superspices. Pour in ¼ cup of water along with taco seasoning and stir frequently to make sure the mix is evenly distributed.

Continue to cook for about five to seven minutes or until done. Remove from heat and let cool. Dice tomato and onion and serve along with shredded cheese, sour cream, and other healthy toppings on my list of recovery superfoods.

Preparation time: Thirty minutes.

STUFFED PEPPERS

INGREDIENTS:

- 1 lb. ground turkey (can substitute ground beef or chicken)
- 3 tbsp. butter
- 1 onion
- 1 tsp. chili powder
- 1 tbsp. chopped parsley
- 4 green peppers
- Sea salt and pepper (to preference)
- 1 tsp. garlic powder (or one clove)
- ½ cup of basmati or whole wheat rice
- 12 oz. or larger can of organic tomato sauce

Preparation: Preheat oven to 325. Brown ground turkey and slowly mix in onions, chili powder, parsley, sea salt, pepper, and garlic. In a separate pot, prepare rice as appropriate (cooking time will vary depending on type of rice you use). Since rice contains carbs, use in moderation with this dinner menu. Once the turkey is browned and all ingredients are mixed well, combine with rice and mix again. Cut off top of peppers and remove seeds and ribs. Fill with mixture and place in a baking dish in the oven. Cover and let cook for one hour.

Preparation time: One hour, thirty minutes.

COOK A FULL TURKEY OR CHICKEN

INGREDIENTS (MULTIPLE SERVINGS):

- One turkey or shicken
- Recovery superspices of your choosing
- Olive oil

Preparation: If turkey or chicken is frozen, defrost thoroughly before cooking. Preheat oven to 375. Wash turkey or chicken well inside and out. Sprinkle spices of your choosing on skin and, to the extent possible, inside. Use olive oil to lubricate the outer skin and avoid burning. Place in preheated oven. Cooking time varies depending on weight. (4 to 8 lbs., cook 1 ½ to 3 ½ hours; 8 to 12 lbs., cook 2 ½ to 4 hours. Freeze what you won't eat right away. A full turkey should last about two weeks.

Preparation time: Time varies.

Healthy Snacks Recipes

POMEGRANATE AVOCADO SALSA

Pomegranate seeds contain fiber, vitamins B6, C, K, folate, potassium, and phosphorous. They are a natural anti-inflammatory, help stabilize blood pressure, fight bacterial infections, and promote heart health. Avocado is one of my recovery superfoods (see Chapter Nine) and is a source of healthy monosaturated fats, fiber, antioxidants, and vitamins B5, B6, C, E, and folate. The healthy fat in an avocado helps to provide energy without spiking blood sugar. Every ingredient in this simple recipe offers a health benefit. Not only is this a healthy choice, but it is absolutely delicious!

INGREDIENTS (THREE SERVINGS):

- 2 cups pomegranates, sliced with seeds removed
- ½ cup of red onion, diced
- ½ cup of chopped fresh cilantro
- 1 jalapeno without seeds and chopped or diced (optional)

- 1 avocado, cut into small chunks
- Lime juice and/or extra-virgin olive oil (amount to your liking)
- 1 tsp. sea salt

Preparation: Mix together pomegranate seeds, red onion, cilantro, jalapeno, and avocado. Fold together gently until everything is mixed together. Mix in sea salt, extra-virgin olive oil, and/or lime juice to taste.

Preparation time: Fifteen minutes.

Low Carb/Glycemic Load Three Bean Salad

INGREDIENTS:

- 12 oz. green string beans
- 12 oz. yellow string beans
- 12 oz. black soy beans
- 1 red pepper
- 1 green pepper
- 1 red onion
- ¼ cup parsley
- Extra-virgin olive oil
- ¼ tsp. garlic powder
- Recovery superspices of your choosing

Preparation: Mix beans into a baking bowl. Then chop peppers and onions and combine with beans. Add extra-virgin olive oil, parsley, and recovery superspices. Mix well and refrigerate. Makes about four servings.

Preparation time: Ten minutes.

Toasted Beet or Sweet Potato Wedge with Fixings

INGREDIENTS:

- 1 sweet potato or beet
- Organic peanut butter
- Honey or other sweetener

- Blueberries (or other fruit of your choosing)
- Recovery superspices of your choosing

Preparation: Cut sweet potato or beet into individual slices (like a bread slice from a loaf of bread). Toast to preference. After toasting, add fixings of your choosing.

Preparation time: Five minutes.

Sweet Potato Fries

INGREDIENTS:

- 1 sweet potato (one per serving)
- Sea salt and black pepper
- Recovery superspices of your choosing.

Preparation: Preheat oven to 275. Cut sweet potato into wedges. Place on baking board and add spices. Bake for five to seven minutes. Turn over and season again. Bake for another three to five minutes.

Preparation time: Ten minutes.

Keto Chili

INGREDIENTS:

- 2 lbs. ultra-lean ground beef (80–90% lean)
- 1 red onion.
- 1 green pepper
- 1 red pepper
- 1 tomato
- 1 6 oz. can organic tomato paste
- Chili spice seasoning (any brand of your choosing as long as all-natural ingredients)
- Sea salt and black pepper (to your preference)
- Recovery superspices of your choosing

Preparation: Brown ground beef and remove excess fat after browning. Finely chop onions, peppers, and tomato and mix into already browned ground beef. Mix in tomato paste, seasoning, and spices and cook on low heat for between eight to fifteen minutes. Stir frequently.

Preparation time: Twenty minutes.

Soup Recipes

CHICKEN VEGETABLE SOUP

INGREDIENTS:

- 1 lb. chicken breast
- Gallon chicken broth
- Veggies of your choosing
- Sea salt and black pepper (to preference)
- Recovery superspices

Preparation: Bake or grill chicken breast until fully cooked. Chop into small cubes or wedges depending on your preference. Chop veggies of your choosing and mix spices in with veggies in a baking bowl. Pour broth into large saucepan. Bring to boil and then reduce to medium heat. Mix in chicken breast, veggies, sea salt, black pepper, and recovery superspices. Cover and cook on medium heat stirring frequently.

Preparation time: Thirty minutes.

Dessert Recipes

FLOURLESS CHOCOLATE CUPCAKES WITH NUTS AND FRUIT

INGREDIENTS:

- 3 oz. dark chocolate (60% and up)
- 2 eggs
- ½ cup butter
- ¼ cup agave or other sweetener
- ⅛ cup filtered water

- 1 cup fruit of your choice
- ¼ cup nuts of your choice

Preparation: Preheat oven to 400, mix agave with water and heat until boiling. Once boiling, remove from heat and add in chocolate. Stir until the chocolate melts. Put back on medium heat and add butter cut in cubes. Continue to stir until all the butter melts (if necessary, lower heat to avoid butter burning). Slowly add beaten eggs and stir until eggs are absorbed into the chocolate mixture. Mix in fruit and nuts and continue to stir until the batter is smooth and consistent, then pour into cupcake molds. Put molds into the preheated oven on a baking sheet (fill each mold half way). Pour water onto the baking dish around the molds. This is known as a "water-bath" and helps to moisturize the mixture. Bake for twenty-five minutes or until mixture expands and fills the cupcake molds. Garnish to your liking.

Preparation time: Forty-five minutes.

Additional substitutions: Organic peanut butter, walnuts, almonds, or other nuts or seeds. You can also incorporate any fruit you like that is in season.

Recommendations: I will cook about a dozen at a time and have them at work and home for healthy snacks.

SWEET POTATO PIE

Turn one of the superfoods, sweet potato, into an amazingly delicious dessert that you won't feel guilty snacking on. Adding nutmeg or cinnamon offers vitamins A, B6, K, niacin, foliate, thiamine, amino acids, powerful antioxidants and anti-inflammatories, and promote heart health while helping to stabilize blood sugar and reduce the chances of type 2 diabetes.

INGREDIENTS (3 SERVINGS):

- 1 pound sweet potato
- ½ teaspoon ground nutmeg
- ½ cup softened butter
- ½ teaspoon ground cinnamon
- ⅔ cup agave

- Alcohol-free pure vanilla extract
- ½ cup skim milk (or soy)
- 1 (9-inch premade graham pie or whole wheat pie crust)
- 2 eggs

Preparation: Boil sweet potato whole in skin for fifty minutes, run cold water over the sweet potato, and remove the skin. Break apart sweet potato in a bowl, add butter, and mix well in a mixer. Stir in agave, milk, eggs, nutmeg, and cinnamon. Mix on medium speed until smooth. Pour filling into an unbaked pie crust. Bake at 350 for sixty minutes or until you can insert a knife into the middle and it comes out clean. When ready, take it out, let it puff up, and then sink down as it cools. Enjoy!

Preparation time: Ninety minutes.

FLAX SEED MUFFINS

INGREDIENTS:

- 1 ½ cups flaxseed meal
- 2 tsp. baking powder
- 1 tbsp. ground cinnamon
- 1 tsp. ground nutmeg
- ½ tsp. salt
- ½ cup applesauce
- 4 eggs beaten
- ¼ cup vegetable oil
- ¼ cup water
- 1 tbsp. vanilla extract
- 1 apple, peeled and chopped
- ½ cup chopped pecans

Preparation: Preheat oven to 350. In a large mixing bowl, mix flaxseed meal, baking powder, cinnamon or nutmeg, and salt. Add applesauce, eggs, oil, ¼ cup water, vanilla, chopped apple, and chopped pecans. Mix thoroughly until all the ingredients are mixed. Let batter settle for ten minutes, portion into cupcake holders. Fill about half way. Put in oven and bake for about eighteen minutes. Keep an eye to avoid burning. It is done when you can insert a toothpick and it comes out clean.

Preparation time: Forty-five minutes.

Beverages Recipes

HOMEMADE SUPERCHARGED DETOX GINGER ALE

Ginger is a powerful antioxidant and among the recovery superfoods. Parsley contains a nutritional punch even in small amounts. One tablespoon has substantial amounts of vitamins A and K, helps to balance your blood sugar, and contains apigenin, a flavonoid that is an anti-inflammatory and antioxidant. The recipe is simple and takes minutes to prepare.

INGREDIENTS:

- Fresh ginger root (one large root)
- Parsley, a handful
- 1 bottle seltzer
- Truvia or another stevia-based natural sweetener (Your preference regarding amount.)

Preparation: Using a cheese shredder, shred one-half cup of ginger root into a wide-mouthed drink container. Mix in small amount of parsley, ⅔ teaspoon of sweetener of your choice, and fill half way with water. Stir well and refrigerate. Prior to drinking, mix half a cup of seltzer water with your premade mix. Make sure to stir the mix well prior to combining with seltzer.

Preparation time: Five minutes.

CINNAMON OR NUTMEG CLEANSE

INGREDIENTS:

- 1 cup almond milk (unsweetened)
- 2 tbsp. of cinnamon
- 2 tbsp. of nutmeg
- Sweetener of your choosing to preference

Preparation: Heat one cup of almond milk slowly. As mixture heats, stir in one tablespoon each of cinnamon and nutmeg. Add any of the recovery sweetener substitutes and stir well. Cool and drink.

Preparation time: Three minutes.

CUMIN, LEMON, FENNEL CLEANSE

INGREDIENTS:

- 2 tsp. cumin
- 2 tsp. fennel
- 1 lemon
- 1 cup water

Preparation: Boil water and when boiling, add the cumin and fennel. Stir well and let sit until it cools. Stir occasionally. Squeeze juice of one fresh lemon into the mixture and stir well. Strain to remove seeds and drink. Add any of the recovery sweetener substitutes and you are good to go either hot or cold.

Preparation time: Three minutes.

TURMERIC GARLIC CLEANSE

INGREDIENTS:

- 1 tsp. turmeric
- 1 tsp. garlic
- 1 cup soy, coconut, almond milk
- Agave or other recovery super sweetener to preference

Preparation: Heat soy, coconut, or almond milk slowly. Once heated, stir in turmeric and garlic. Stir well while heating. Remove from heat, let cool, and stir in recovery super sweetener to your preference.

Preparation time: Five minutes.

Notes

CHAPTER ONE

1 M. Miller, "The Relevance of Twelve-Step Recovery in 21st Century Addiction Medicine," American Society of Addiction Medicine, https://www.asam.org/resources/publications/magazine/read/article/2015/02/13/the-relevance-of-twelve-step-recovery-in-21st-century-addiction-medicine, accessed February 13, 2015.

2 Theodore Ficken, "Music Therapy with Chemically Dependent Clients: A Relapse Prevention Model," *Music Therapy and Addictions* (2012): 110.

3 Ibid., 109.

4 A. Paoli, "Beyond Weight Loss: A review of the therapeutic uses of very-low-carbohydrate (ketogenic) diets," *European Journal of Clinical Nutrition* 67, no. 8 (2013): 789–96.

5 L. P. Grant, B. Haughton, and D. S. Sachan, "Nutrition Education Is Positively Associated with Substance Abuse Treatment Program Outcomes," *Journal of the American Dietetic Association* 104, no. 4 (2004): 604–10.

6 Katherine Ketcham and L. Ann Mueller, *Eating Right to Live Sober* (Writers House Publishing, 1986), 78–79.

7 Ibid., 165.

8 Beth Reardon, "Are There Foods That Will Help with Withdrawal Symptoms of an Opiate Addiction," Duke Integrative Medicine, www.caring.com, https://www.caring.com/questions/foods-that-help-with-opiate-withdrawal.

9 M. S. Westerterp-Plantenga, "Protein Intake and Energy Balance," *Regulatory Peptides* 149, no. 1–3 (2008): 67–69.

10 N. M. Avena, P. Rada, B. G. Hoebel, "Evidence for Sugar Addiction: Behavioral and Neurochemical Effects of Intermittent, Excessive Sugar Intake," *Neuroscience & Biobehavioral Review* 32, no. 1 (2008): 20–39.

11 Jimmy Moore and Eric C. Westman, *Keto Clarity, Your Definitive Guide to the Benefits of A Low-Carb, High-Fat Diet* (Las Vegas, NV: Victory Belt Publishing, 2014).

12 Bill P., Todd W. and Sara S., *Drop the Rock: Removing Character Defects, Second Edition* (Minneapolis, MN: Hazelden Foundation, 2005), 29.

13 M. Blum, et al., "The Molecular Neurobiology of Twelve Steps Program & Fellowship: Connecting the Dots for Recovery," *Journal of Reward Deficiency Syndrome* 1, no. 1 (2015), 46–64.

14 Ibid., 2.

15 Ibid., 12.

16 Ibid., 13.

17 M. Galanter, "An initial fMRI study on neural correlates of prayer in members of Alcoholics Anonymous," *American Journal of Drug and Alcohol Abuse* 43, no. 1 (2017).

18 C. L. Robertson, et al., "Effect of Exercise Training on Striatal Dopamine D2/D3 Receptors in Methamphetamine Users during Behavioral Treatment," *Neuropsychopharmacology* 41 (2016): 1629–36.

CHAPTER TWO

19 Alcoholics Anonymous, *Dr. Bob and the Good Oldtimers* (New York: A.A. World Services, Inc., 1980), 80.

20 Alcoholics Anonymous, '*Pass It On*': *The Story of Bill Wilson and How the A.A. Message Reached the World* (New York: A.A. World Services, Inc., 1984), 388–89.

21 What is now known as Type 2 diabetes was not prevalent at the time among children and young adults. As the amount of sugar in the common diet has increased, diabetes acquired through poor nutrition began to impact younger demographics, including young children. Accordingly, the name was changed to reflect this societal change.

22 J. D. Beasley and S. Knightly, *Food for Recovery*, (New York: Crown Trade Publishing, 1993), 53.

23 Ibid., 53.

24 A. Hoffer and A. Saul, *The Vitamin Cure to Alcoholism* (Laguna Beach, CA: Basic Health Publications, 2008), 23–25.

25 *Alcoholics Anonymous Co-Founder Bill Wilson Used Niacin to Stop Alcoholism*, June 17, 2011, www.stop-alcohol27.blogspot.com.

26 Joan Mathews Larson, *Seven Weeks to Sobriety* (New York: First Ballantine Books, 1997), citing research conducted by Emanuel Cheraskin, "Consequences of Alcohol Use in Diabetics," *Alcohol Health & Research World* 22, no. 3 (1998): 211–19.

27 J. Farres, "Revealing the molecular relationship between type 2 diabetes and the metabolic changes induced by a very-low-carbohydrate low-fat ketogenic diet," *Nutrition and Metabolism* 7, no. 1 (2010): 1–9.

28 M. Poplawski, et al., "Reversal of Diabetic Nephropathy by a Ketogenic Diet," *PLoS One* 6, no. 4 (2011): E18604.

29 *Snuffing Out Tobacco in the Recovery Community*, The Voice, Hazelton Betty Ford Foundation (2002).

CHAPTER THREE

30 Bill P., Todd W. and Sara S, *Drop the Rock*, 38.

31 P. Rada, N. M. Avenua, and B. G. Hoebel, "Daily Bingeing on Sugar Repeatedly Releases Dopamine in the Accumbens Shell," *Neuroscience* 134, no. 3 (2005): 737–44.

32 G. DiChiara and V. Bassareo, "Reward System and Addiction: What Dopamine Does and Doesn't Do," *Pharmacology* 7, no. 2 (2007): 233.

33 J. R. Milam and K. Ketcham, *Under the Influence* (New York: Bantam Books, 1983), 28.

34 Ibid., 29.

35 Ibid., 29.

36 M. J. Foley, *Eat To Be Fit* (Portland, ME: Living Well Publishing Company, 2002), 9.

37 J. C. Martin, *Chalk Talk* (New York: Harper Collins, 1973), 11–16.

38 M. Yen and M. Ewald, "Toxicity of Weight Loss Agents," *Journal of Medical Toxicology* 8, no. 2 (2012): 145–52.

39 D. Mysels and M. Sullivan, "The Relationship Between Opioid and Sugar Intake: Review of Evidence and Clinical Applications," *Journal of Opioid Management* 6, no. 6 (2010): 445–52.

40 K. Ketcham and L. A. Mueller, *Eating Right to Live Sober* (Writers House Publishing, 1986).

41 M. E. Van Eiswyk and S. H. McNeil, "Impact of grass/forage feeding versus grain finishing on beef nutrients and sensory quality: The U.S. experience," *Meat Science*, 96, no. 1 (2014), 535–40.

42 E. J. DePeters, "Can fatty acid and mineral compositions of sturgeon eggs distinguish between farm-raised versus wild white (Acipenser transmontanus) sturgeon origins in California? Preliminary Report," *Forensic Science International* 229, no. 1–3 (2013): 126–32.

43 S. Leclercq, et al, "The link between inflammation, bugs, the intestine and the brain in alcohol dependence," *Translational Psychiatry* 7, no. 2 (2017): E1048.

44 H. Kolb, "The global diabetes epidemic as a consequence of lifestyle-induced low-grade inflammation," *Diabetologia* 53, no. 1 (2010): 10–20.

45 L. M. Coussens and Z. Werb, "Inflammation and Cancer," *Nature* (2002): 860–67.

46 B. S. Lennerz, et al., "Effects of dietary glycemic index on brain regions related to reward and cravings in men," *The American Journal of Clinical Nutrition* 98, no. 3 (2013): 641–47.

47 C. Olsen, "Natural Rewards, Neuroplasticity, and Non-Drug Addictions," *Neuropharmacology* 61, no. 7 (2011): 1109–22.

48 *Eating Right to Live Sober*, (Writers House Publishing, 1986), 165.

49 Lieber S. Charles, *Medical and Nutritional Complications of Alcoholism, Mechanism and Management* (New York: Plenum Publishing Corporation, 1992), 517.

50 *The Psychology of Carbohydrate Addiction and Why it Makes Us Fat,* (February 20, 2014).

51 Ibid., *see also* N. M. Avena, "Evidence for sugar addiction: behavioral and neurochemical effects of intermittent, excessive sugar intake," *Neuroscience and Biobehavioral Reviews* 32 (2007): 20–39.

52 Sue Brown, *Simply Sugar Free*, (Promoting Natural Health, LLC, 2014), 11.

53   Ibid., 12.

54   Ibid., 14.

55   B. S. Lennerz, et al., "Effects of dietary glycemic index on brain regions related to reward and craving in men," *The American Journal of Clinical Nutrition*, 98, no 3 (2013): 641–47.

56   Sue Brown, *Simply Sugar Free* (Promoting Natural Health, LLC, 2014), 19.

57   M. S. Westerterp-Plantenga, "Protein Intake and Energy Balance," *Regulatory Peptides* 149, no. 1–3 (2008): 67–9. www.ncbi.nlm.nlh.gov/pubmed/18448177.

58   M. A. Veldhorst, et al, "Presence or absence of carbohydrates and the proportion of fat in a high-protein diet affect appetite suppression but not energy expenditure in normal-weight human subjects fed in energy balance," *British Journal of Nutrition* 104 (2010), 1395–1405.

59   Beasley and Knightly, *Food for Recovery*, 21.

CHAPTER FOUR

60   L. Cordain, S. B. Eaton, A. Sebastian, et al. "Origins and Evolution of the Western Diet: Health implications for the 21st Century," *American Journal Clinical Nutrition* 81 (2005), 341–54.

61   D. A. Roe, "Drugs and Nutrient Absorption," *Current Concepts in Nutrition* 12 (1983): 129–38.

62   J. P. Bonjour, "Vitamins and Alcoholism," *International Journal of Vitamin and Nutrition Research* 51 (1981): 166–77.

63   Charles S. Lieber, *Medical and Nutritional Complications of Alcoholism: Mechanisms and Management* (New York: Medical Book Company, 1992), 515.

64   Ibid., 516–18.

65   G. J. Tortora, N. P. Anagnostakos, *Principles of Anatomy and Physiology*, *Fifth Edition* (New York: Harper & Row Publishers, 1987).

66   E. L. Burnham, "The Relationship Between Airway Antioxidant Levels, Alcohol Use Disorders, and Cigarette Smoking," *Alcoholism Clinical and Experimental Research* 40, no. 10 (2016): 2147–60.

67   S. Nabipour, M. Ayu Said, M. Hussain Habil, "Burden and Nutritional Deficiencies in Opiate Addiction– Systematic Review Article," *Iran Journal of Public Health* 43, no. 8 (2014): 1022–32.

68   Ibid., 5.

69   D. J. Mysels, et al., "The relationship between opioid and sugar intake: Review of evidence and clinical applications," *Journal of Opioid Management* 6, no. 6 (2010): 445–52.

70   K. Ersche, "The skinny on cocaine: Insights into eating behavior and body weight in cocaine-dependent men," *Appetite* 71 (2013): 75–80.

71   Roberta Andin, MS, RD, spokesperson for the American Dietetic Association, www.webmd.com/vitamins-and-supplements/nutrition-vitamins-11/help-vitamin-supplement; Kathleen M. Zelman, "What Vitamin and Mineral Supplements Can and Can't Do," *Balanced Living News*, http://www.balancedlivingnews.com/topic/profile/kathleen-m-zelman/.

72   www.cavemandoctor.com.

73   Caveman Doctor, "Stop Pills and Eat Your Vitamins and Nutrients," 2012, 6, www.cavemandoctor.com, citing S. M. Zhang, N. R. Cook, C. M. Albert, et al.,

"Effect of folic acid, Vitamin B6, and Vitamin B12 on cancer risk in women, a randomized trial," *Journal of the American Medical Association* 300 (2008): 2012–21; "Dietary supplementation with n-3 polyunsaturated fatty acids and vitamin E after myocardial infarction: results of the GISSI-Prevenzion trial. Gruppo Italiano per lo Studio della Sopravvivensza nell'infanto myocardico," *Lancet* 354, no. 9177 (1999): 447–55; K. G. Joshipura, F. B. Hu, J. E. Manson, et al., "The Effect of Fruit and Vegetable Intake on Risk for Coronary Heart Disease," *Annals of Internal Medicine* 134 (2001): 1106–14; S. M. Lippman, E. A. Klein, P. J. Goodman, et al., "Effect of Selenium and Vitamin E on Risk of Prostate Cancer and Other Cancers," *Journal of the American Medical Association* 301 (2009): 39–51.

74   E. O'Connor, "Vitamin D-vitamin K interaction: effect of vitamin D supplementation on serum percentage undercarboxylated osteocalcin, a sensitive measure of vitamin K status, in Danish girls," *British Journal of Nutrition* 104, no. 8 (2010): 1091–95; *see also* A. Arnarson, "Is vitamin D harmful without vitamin K," *Authority Nutrition*, (2017), www.authoritynutrition.com/vitamin-d-and-vitamin-k.; E. L. Burnham, "The Relationship Between Airway Antioxidant Levels, Alcohol Use Disorders, and Cigarette Smoking," *Alcoholism, Clinical and Experimental Research* 40, no. 10 (2016): 2147–60, Epub 2016 (2016): 2147–60.

75   O. Arias-Carrión, et al., "Dopaminergic reward system: a short integrative review," *International Archives of Medicine* 3 (2010): 24.

76   Y. Kim, Y. Je, "Flavonoid intake and mortality from cardiovascular disease and all causes: A meta-analysis of prospective cohort studies," *Clinical Nutrition ESPEN* 20 (2017): 68–77.

77   M. Doi, I. Yamaoka, T. Fukunaga, M. Nakayama, "Isoleucine, a potent plasma glucose-lowering amino acid, stimulates glucose uptake in C2C12 myotubes," *Biochemical and Biophysical Research Communication* 312, no. 4 (2003): 1111–7.

78   E. L. Metcaslfe, A. Avenell, A. Fraser, "Branched-chain amino acid supplementation in adults with cirrhosis and port-systemic encephalopathy: systematic review," *Clinical Nutrition* 33, no. 6 (2014): 958–65.

79   *Seven Weeks*, 106.

CHAPTER FIVE

80   J. Gy, et al., "Effect of aerobic exercise and resistance exercise in improving non-alcoholic fatty liver disease: a randomized controlled trial," *Chinese Journal of Hepatology* 26, no. 1 (2018), 34–41; C. Poblete-Aro, "Exercise and oxidative stress in type 2 diabetes mellitus," *Revista Medica de Chile* 146, no. 3 (2016): 362–72; C. Fu, et al., "Effects of rehabilitation exercise on coronary artery after percutaneous coronary intervention in patient with coronary heart disease: a systematic review and meta-analysis," *Disability and Rehabilitation* 10 (2018): 1–7.

81   L. S. Robison, et al., "Exercise Reduces Dopamine D1R and Increases D2R in Rats: Implications for Addiction," *Medicine and Science in Sports and Medicine* 50, no. 8 (2018): 1596–1602; M. A. Smith, et al., "Resistance exercise decreases heroin self-administration and alters gene expression in the nucleus accumbens of heroin-exposed rats," *Psycholpharmacology* 235, no. 4, 1245–55 (2018).

82   National Institute on Drug Abuse, "Misuse of Prescription Drugs," August 2016, 1; *see also* The Dawn Report, *Highlights of the 2010 Drug Abuse Warning Network Findings on Drug-Related Emergency Department Visits* (July 2012).

83   Fred H., *The Ripple Effect: Using Step 10 to Work Steps 6 and 7 Every Day* (Minneapolis, MN: Hazelden Publishing, 2016), 78.

84   J. P. Read, et al., "Exercise attitudes and behaviors among person in treatment for alcohol use disorders," *Journal of Substance Abuse Treatment* 21 (2001): 199–206.

85   Ibid., 7.

86   A. H. Taylor, et al., "Acute effect of exercise on alcohol urges and attentional bias towards alcohol related images in high alcohol consumers," *Mental Health and Physical Activity* 6, no. 3 (2013), 220–26.

87   Ibid., 225–26.

88   M. S. Buchowski, et al., "Aerobic exercise training reduces cannabis cravings and use in non-treatment seeking cannabis-dependent adults," *PLoS One* 6, no. 3 (2011): e.17465.

89   R. A. Brown, et al, "A pilot study of aerobic exercise as an adjunctive treatment for drug dependence," *Mental Health and Physical Activity* 3 (2010): 27–34.

90   E. J. Barbanti, "The Effects of Simple Exercise on Life of Patients Suffering From Depression," *Revista Brasileira de Atividade Fisica & Saude* 11, (2006): 37–45.

91   Ibid., 43–45.

92   B. N. Greenwood, *et al.,* "Long-term voluntary wheel running is rewarding and produces plasticity in the mesolimbic reward pathway," *Behavioural Brain Research* 217, no. 2 (2011): 354–62.

93   S. Stroth, et al., "Impact of aerobic exercise training on cognitive functions and effect associated to the COMT polymorphism in young adults," *Neurobiology of Learning and Memory* 94, no. 3 (2010): 364–72, cited by K. Blum, S. Teitelbaum, M. Oscar, *Molecular Neurobiology of Addiction Recovery: The 12 Steps Program and Fellowship* (New York: Springer Publications, 2013): 26.

94   J. L. Medina, et al., "Exercise and coping-oriented alcohol use among a trauma exposed sample," *Addictive Behaviors* 36 (2011): 274–77.

95   Ibid., 275.

96   Ibid.

97   J. Weinstock, et al., "Exercise-related activities are associated with positive outcome in contingency management treatments for substance abuse disorders," *Addictive Behaviors* 33 (2008): 1072–75.

98   Ibid., 1274–75.

99   Ibid.

100 M. Ussher, et al., "Acute Effect of a brief bout of exercise on alcohol urges," *Addiction* 99, no. 12 (2004): 1542–47 *see also* L. F. Costa Rosa, "Exercise as a time-conditioning effector in chronic disease: A complimentary treatment strategy," *Evidence-based Complementary and Alternative Medicine* 1 (2004): 63–70.

101 R. De La Garza, et al., "Treadmill exercise improves fitness and reduces craving and use of cocaine in individuals with concurrent cocaine and tobacco-use disorder," *Psychiatry Research* 245 (2016): 133–140.

102 C. L. Robertson, et al., "Effect of Exercise Training on Striatal Dopamine D2/D3 Receptors in Methamphetamine Users during Behavior Treatment," *Neuropsycholpharmacology* 41 (2016): 1629–36.

CHAPTER SIX

103 B. Wilson, *As Bill Sees It,* (New York: A.A. Publications), 184.

104 M. Beattie, *The Language of Letting Go* (Minneapolis, MN: Hazelden Foundation Press, 1990), 105.

105 N. Zitron-Emanuel, "The effect of food deprivation on human resolving powers," *Psychonomic Bulletin and Review* 25, no. 1 (2017): 455–62.

106 *Just For Today: Daily Meditations for Recovery Addicts,* (Van Nuys, CA: Narcotics Anonymous, 1991), 156.

107 Ibid.

108 B. Wilson, *As Bill Sees It* (New York: A.A. Publications), 90.

109 D. A. Almbach, "Sleep Disturbances and Short Sleep as Risk Factors for Depression and Perceived Medical Errors in First-Year Residents," *Sleep* 40, no. 3 (2017); M. Kragh, "Wake and light therapy for moderate-to-severe depression–a randomized controlled trial," *Acta Psychiatrica Scandinavica* 136, no. 6 (2017): 559–70.

CHAPTER SEVEN

110 L. J. Vanderschuren, et al., "Sensitization processes in drug addiction," *Current Topics in Behavioral Neurosciences* 3 (2010): 179–85.

111 T. E. Robinson, K. C. Berridge, "The neural basis of drug craving: an incentive-sensitization theory of addiction," *Brain Research, Brain Research Reviews* 18, no. 3 (1993): 247–91.

112 https://www.niaid.nih.gov/diseases-conditions/guidelines-clinicians-and-patients-food-allergy

113 P. Begin, et al., "Natural resolution of peanut allergy: a 12-year longitudinal follow-up study," *Journal of Allergy and Clinical Immunology: In Practice* 1, no. 5 (2013): 528–30.

114 S. Currie, et al., "Alcohol Induces Sensitization to Gluten in Genetically Susceptible Individuals: A Case Control Study," *PLoS One* 8, no. 10 (2013): E77638. *See also* R. Bradunaie, "Influence of alcohol consumption on the autoimmune process," *Acta Medica Lituanica* 9 (2002): 245–57; D. J. Meyerhoff, "Effects of heavy drinking, binge drinking, and family history of alcoholism on regional brain metabolites," *Alcoholism Clinical and Experimental Research* 28 (2004): 650–61.

115 Ibid., 246.

116 B. Wilson, *Alcoholics Anonymous, Second Edition* (New York: A.A. World Services), 67.

117 S. N. Seidman, "Testosterone deficiency and mood in aging men: pathogenic and therapeutic interactions," *The World Journal of Biological Psychiatry* 4, no. 1 (2003): 14–20.

118 Suzy Cohen, *Drug Muggers: Which Medications Are Robbing Your Body of Essential Nutrients–and Natural Ways to Restore Them* (New York: Rodale Publishing, 2011), 7.

119 Ibid., 23–63.

120 A. Hansen, *Five experts on whether BMI is a useful indicator of health,* Sydney Morning Herald, Health & Wellness Section (July 4, 2018).

121 Narcotics Anonymous, *Just for Today, Sixth Edition,* (Narcotics Anonymous World Services: Van Nuys, CA. (2013), 135.

122 Ibid.

CHAPTER EIGHT

123 H. R. Rabinovitz, et al.,"Big Breakfast rich in protein and fat improves glycemic control in type 2 diabetes," *Obesity* 22, no. 5 (2014): E46–E54.

124 Ibid., *see also* Kathleen DesMaisons, *Potatoes Not Prozac* (New York: Simon & Schuster, 1998), 74–75.

125 Ibid., *see also* Kathleen DesMaisons, *Potatoes Not Prozac*, 92.

126 H. R. Rabinovitz, "Big Breakfast rich in protein and fat improves glycemic control in type 21 diabetes," *Obesity* 22, no. 5 (May 2014): E46–E54.

127 J. Anderson and C. Fitzgerald, *Iron: An Essential Nutrient*, June 2010.

128 Ibid.

129 M. Ritu, "Nutritional composition of Stevia rebaudiana, a sweet herb, and its hypoglycemic and hypolipidemic effect on patients with non-insulin dependent diabetes mellitus," *Journal of the Science of Food and Agriculture* (2016), 4231–4.

130 I. Aranda-Gonzalez, et al., "Evaluation of the Antihyperglycemic Effect of Minor Steviol Glycosides in Normoglycemic and Induced-Diabetic Wistar Rats," *Journal of Medicinal Food* 19, no. 9 (2016): 844–52.

131 C. L. Chukuma and M. S. Islam, "Effects of xylitol on carbohydrate digesting enzymes activity, intestinal glucose absorption and muscle glucose uptake: a multi-mode study," *Food and Function* 3 (2015): 955–62; M. S. Islam, M. Indraijit, "Effects of xylitol on blood glucose, glucose intolerance, serum insulin and lipid profile in a type 2 diabetes model of rats," *Annals of Nutrition and Metabolism* 61, no. 1 (2012): 57–64; S. Ur-Rehman, et al., "Xylitol: a review on bioproduction, application, health benefits, and related safety issues," *Critical Reviews in Food Science and Nutrition* 55, no. 11 (2015): 1514–28.

132 Nutrition Action, "Sweet Nothings, Safe . . . or scary?: The Inside Scoop on Sugar Substitutes," November 12, 2014.

133 Ibid.

134 P. Humphries, E. Pretorius, and H. Naude, "Direct and indirect cellular effects of aspartame on the brain," Department of Anatomy, University of Pretoria, Gauteng, South African and University of Limpopo, South Africa, October 24, 2006.

135 P. Humphries, E. Pretorius, and H. Naude, "Direct and Indirect Cellular Effects of Aspartame on the Brain," *European Journal of Clinical Nutrition* 62, no. 4 (2008): 451–62.

136 G. Naveed Sattar, "Fruit Juice, Just Another Sugary Drink?" *The Lancet Diabetes & Endocrinology* 2, no. 6 (2014): 444–46.

137 Shrinivas Kulkarni, et al., "*Potentials of Curcumin as an Antidepressant*," (Chandigarh, India: Pharmacology Division, University Institute of Pharmaceutical Sciences, Panjab University), October 16, 2009; Shrinivas Kulkarni et al., "Antidepressant Activity of Curcumin: Involvement of Serotonin and Dopamine Systems," *Psychopharmacology* 201 (2008): 435–42; Y. Xu, et al., "The Effects of Curcumin on Depressive-Like Behaviors in Mice," *European Journal of Pharmacology* 518 (2005): 40–46.

138 Nafiseh Khandouzi, et al., "The Effects of Ginger on Fasting Blood Sugar, Hemoglobin A1c, Apolipoprotein B, Apolipoprotein A-1, and Malondialdehyde in Type 2 Diabetic Patients," *Iranian Journal of Pharmaceutical Research* 14, no. 1 (2015): 131–40.

139 Pasupuleti Visweswara Rao and Siew Hau Gan, *Cinnamon: A Multifaceted Medicinal Plant, Journal of Evidence Based Complimentary and Alternative Medicine*,

April 10, 2014. Available online at www.ncbi.nlm.gov/pmc/articles/PMC 4003790.

140 A. Khan, M. Safdar, et al., "Cinnamon Improves Glucose and Lipids of People with Type 2 Diabetes," *Diabetes Care* 26, no. 12 (2003): 3215–18; B. Qin, et al, "Cinnamon: Potential Role in the Prevention of Insulin Resistance, Metabolic Syndrome of Type 2 Diabetes," *Journal of Diabetes Science and Technology* 4, no. 3 (2010): 685–93; S. Kirkham, "The Potential of Cinnamon to Reduce Blood Glucose Levels in Patients with Type 2 Diabetes and Insulin Resistance," *Diabetes Obesity & Metabolism* 11, no. 12 (2009): 1100–13; A. Q. Pham, et al., "Cinnamon Supplementation in Patients With Type 2 Diabetes Mellitus," *Pharmacotherapy* 27, no 4 (2007): 595–99.

141 C. Kuo, C. Chi, and T. Liu, "The Anti-Inflammatory Potential of Berberine In Vitro and In Vivo," *Cancer Letters* 203, no. 2 (2004): 127–37.

142 H. Zhang, "Berberine Lowers Blood Glucose in Type 2 Diabetes Mellitus Patients through Increasing Insulin Receptor Expression," *Journal Metabolism* 59, no. 2 (2010): 285–92.

143 X. Xia et al., "Berberine Improves Glucose Metabolism in Diabetic Rats by Inhibition of Hepatic Gluconeogenesis," *PLoS One* 6, no. 2 (2011): e16556.

144 J. Yin, H. Zhang, and J. Ye, "Traditional Chinese Medicine in Treatment of Metabolic Syndrome," *Journal Metabolism* 8, no. 2 (2008): 99–111; Y. Wang, et al., "Synthesis and Biological Evaluation of Berberine Analogues as Novel Up-Regulators for Both Low-Density Lipoprotein Receptor and Insulin Receptor," *Bioorganic & Medicinal Chemistry Letters* 19, no. 21 (2009): 6004–8.

145 X. Chang, et al., "Berberine Reduces Methylation of the MTTP Promoter and Alleviates Fatty Liver Induced by a High-Fat Diet in Rats," *Journal of Lipid Research* 51, no. 9 (2010): 2504–15.

146 X. Sun, et al., "Berberine Inhibits Hepatic Stellate Cell Proliferation and Prevents Experimental Liver Fibrosis," *Biological & Pharmaceutical Bulletin* 32, no. 9 (2009): 1533–37.

147 J. Borlinghaus et al., "Allicin: Chemistry and Biological Properties," *Molecules* 19, no. 8 (2014): 12591–618;
Karin Ried, et al., "Effect of Garlic on Blood Pressure: A Systematic Review and Meta-Analysis," *BMC Cardiovascular Disorders* 8 (2008): 13; R. Ashraf, et al., "Effects Of Allium Sativum (Garlic) on Systolic and Diastolic Blood Pressure in Patients with Essential Hypertension" *Pakistan Journal of Pharmaceutical Sciences* (2013): 859–63.

148 M. Moss, *Are Nuts a Weight-Loss Aid?* (Lafayette, IN: Purdue University, 2013).

149 *Recovery2.0, supra*, pg. 251, 252.

150 A. O'Connor, "Caffeine-Laced Foods Spur F.D.A. Investigation," *New York Times*, May 3, 2013.

151 Ibid.

CHAPTER NINE

152 Citations are omitted as these issues are addressed earlier in the chapter.

153 A. Paoli, et al., "Beyond weight loss: a review of the therapeutic uses of very-low-carbohydrate (ketogenic) diets," *European Journal of Clinical Nutrition* 67, no 8 (2013): 789–96.

154 S. K. Raatz, "Consumption of Honey, Sucrose, and High-Fructose Corn Syrup Produces Similar Metabolic Effects in Glucose-Tolerant and Intolerant Individuals," *The Journal of Nutrition* 145 (2015): 2265–72.

155 M. Chung, et al., "Fructose, high-fructose corn syrup, sucrose, and nonalcoholic fatty liver disease or indexes of liver health: a systematic review and meta-analysis," *American Journal of Clinical Nutrition* 100 (2014): 833–49.

156 D. De Stefanis, "Effects of chronic sugar consumption on lipid accumulation and autophagy in the skeletal muscle," *European Journal of Nutrition* 56 (2017): 363–73.

157 C. S. Lieber, et al., "Difference in Hepatic Metabolism of Long and Medium-Chain Fatty Acids: the Role of Fatty Acid Chain Length in the Production of the Alcoholic Fatty Liver," *The Journal of Clinical Investigation* 46 (1967): 1451–60.

158 M. P. St.-Onge and P. Jones, "Physiological Effects of Medium-Chain Triglycerides: Potential Agents in the Prevention of Obesity," *The Journal of Nutrition* 132, no. 3 (2002): 329–32.

159 Paoli, A., et al., "Beyond Weight Loss: A Review of the Therapeutic Uses of Very-low-carbohydrate (ketogenic) diets," *European Journal of Clinical Nutrition* 67, no. 8 (2013): 789–96.

160 Ibid.

161 M. Ahmed, "Non-alcoholic fatty liver disease in 2015," *World Journal of Hepatology* 7 (2015): 1450–59.

162 Ibid.

163 Ibid., *see also What is Fatty Liver?* www.doctortipser.com/25755-fatty-liver-and-obesity.html.

164 Ibid., *see also* K. D. Fairbanks, *Alcoholic Liver Disease,* www.clevelandclinicmeded.com.

165 "Alcoholic Liver Disease (ALD)," www.webmd.com.

166 X. Shi, "Lipidomic profiling reveals protective function of fatty acid oxidation in cocaine-inducted hepatotoxicity," *Journal of Lipid Research* 53, no. 11 (2011): 2318–30.

167 Ibid., *see also* H. Volzke, "Multicausality in fatty liver disease: Is there a rationale to distinguish between alcoholic and non-alcoholic origin?" *World Journal of Gastroenterology* 18 (2012): 3492–3501.

168 Ibid.

169 J. F. Vettorazzi, et al., "The bile acid TUDCA increases glucose-induced insulin secretion via the cAMP/PKA pathway in pancreatic beta cells," *Metabolism* 65, no. 3 (2016) 54–63; E. A. Tsochatzis, "Liver cirrhosis," *Lancet* 383 (2014) 1749–61; A. Crosignani, "Tauroursodeoxycholic acid for the treatment of HCV-related chronic hepatitis: a multicenter placebo-controlled study," *Hepatogastroenterology* 45 (1998) 1624–29; M. Kars, "Tauroursodeoxycholic Acid may improve liver and muscle but not adipose tissue insulin sensitivity in obese men and women," *Diabetes* 59 (2010): 1899–1905; U. Ozcan, "Endoplasmic reticulum stress links obesity, insulin action, and type 2 diabetes," *Science* 306 (2004) 457–61.

170 A. Genoni, et al., "Cardiovascular, Metabolic Effects, and Dietary Composition of Ad-Libitum Paleolithic vs. Australian Guide to Healthy Eating Diets: A 4-Week Randomised Trial," *Nutrients* 8, no. 5 (2016): E314; R. L. Pastore, et al., "Paleolithic nutrition improves plasma lipid concentrations of hypercholesterolemic adults to a greater extent than traditional heart-healthy dietary recommendations," *Nutritional Research* 35, no. 6 (2015): 474–79; P. M. Ryan, "Functional food addressing heart

health: do we have to target the gut microbiota?" *Current Opinion in Clinical Nutritional Metabolic Care* 18, no. 6 (2015): 566–71.

171 BUN refers to the amount of nitrogen in your blood. The higher the amount of nitrogen, the less effectively the body is eliminating toxins. Extremely high BUN levels can result in organ failure over time.

172 L. G. Boros, et al., "Ethanol diversely alters palmitate, stearate and oleate metabolism in the liver and pancreas of rats using the deuterium oxide single tracer," *Pancreas* 38 (2009): 47–52, *see also* http://www.drweil.com/drw/u/ART03144/Pancreatitis.html

173 Ibid.

174 Ibid.

175 Christine Gerbstadt, *Doctor's Detox Diet: The Ultimate Weight Loss Prescription* (NUTRONICS, 2012).

176 P. Rose, et al, "Broccoli and watercress suppress matrix metalloproteinase-9 activity and invasiveness of human MDA-MB-231 breast cancer cells," *Toxicology and Applied Pharmacology* 209 (2005): 105–113; *see also* H. Steinkellner, et al., "Effects of cruciferous vegetables and their constituents on drug metabolizing enzymes involved in the bioactivation of DNA-reactive dietary carcinogens," *Mutation Research* 480–481 (2001): 285–97.

177 Ibid.

CHAPTER TEN

178 J. Pilates, *Pilates' Return to Life Through Contrology: Revised Edition for the 21st Century* (Pompano Beach, FL: Presentation Dynamics, 2012).

179 A. Schwarzenegger, *The New Encyclopedia of Modern Bodybuilding: The Bible of Bodybuilding* (New York: Simon & Schuster, 1998), xxii.

180 https://www.crossfit.com/what-is-crossfit.

181 J. C. Herz, *Learning to Breathe Fire, The Rise of Crossfit and the Primal Future of Fitness* (New York: Three Rivers Press, 2014), 13.

182 R. S. Mishra, *The Textbook of Yoga Psychology, A Definitive Translation & Interpretation of the Yoga Sutras of Patanjali* (New York: The Julian Press, 1987), xii.

183 *The Yoga Sutras of Patanjali, Fourth Edition*, Translation and Commentary by Sri Swami Satchidananda, (Buckingham, VA, Integral Yoga Publications, 2015).

184 Ibid., Introduction, xi.

185 Ibid.

186 T.K.V., Desikachar, *Heart of Yoga: Developing A Personal Practice* (Rochester, VT: Inner Traditions International, 1999).trition to you are looking to leost impossible to ustlce. e point is that you must vary your nutrition to you are looking to le

187 Siler, B., *The Pilates Body, First Edition* (New York: Harmony Books, 2007).

188 Ibid., pg. 7.

189 Ibid., pg. 15.

190 Ibid.

191 https://y12sr.com/about/.

192 Moreno, P., The intenSati Method, *Simon Spotlight Entertainment*, (2009), 3.

193 Ibid., 5.

194 https://thephoenix.org/about/.

195 The Phoenix, *Impact Report*, December 2017.

196 *Evaluation of the Addicts to Athletes Programs*, Center for Research Strategies, 10th Judicial District, Probation Department (2016).

197 http://www.addict2athlete.org/.

198 https://www.rocoveryfitness.org/

199 T. Rosen, *Recovery2.0: Move Beyond Addiction and Upgrade Your Life* (Carlsbad, CA: Hay House, Inc., 2014), 11.

200 J. Thompson Coon, "Does Participating in Physical Activity in Outdoor Natural Environments Have a Greater Effect on Physical and Mental Wellbeing than Physical Activity Indoors? A Systematic Review," *Environmental Science and Technology* 45 (2011): 1761–72.

201 J. O. Barron and J. Pretty, "What is the Best Dose of Nature and Green Exercise for Improving Mental Health? A Multi-Study Analysis," *Environmental Science and Technology* 44 (2010): 3947–55.

202 A. M. Abrantes, et al., "Developing a Fitbit-supported lifestyle physical activity intervention for depressed alcohol dependent women," *Journal of Substance Abuse Treatment* 80 (2017): 88–97.

203 Ibid.

204 Ibid.

205 V. N. Mishra, et al., "Exercise Beyond Menopause: Dos and Don'ts," *Journal of Midlife Health* (2011): 51–56.

206 *Eat to Be Fit*, 93.

207 S.A. Bobzean, et al., "Sex Differences in the neurobiology of drug addiction," *Experimental Neurology* 259 (2014): 64–74.

208 C. A. Hernandez-Avila, "Opiod-, cannabis- and- alcohol dependent women show more rapid progression to substance abuse treatment," *PlumX Metrics* 74, no. 3 (2004): 265–72.

209 C. Ortega, Rise and Grind program helps local women in recovery, KOLO-TV, Reno, April 25, 2018.

210 http://www.ktvn.com/story/37441388/rise-grind-program-helps-area-women-in-recovery.

CHAPTER ELEVEN

211 *Alcoholics Anonymous*, A.A. World Services, 83.

212 P. Stutz, and B. Michels, *The Tools: Transform Your Problems Into Courage, Confidence and Creativity*, (New York: Spiegel & Grau, 2012).

213 Ibid., 6.

214 Ibid., 15.

215 Ibid., 19.

216 J. Pilates, *Pilates' Return to Life Through Contrology* (1945): 24.

217 A. Alter, *Irresistible: The Rise of Addictive Technology and the Business of Keeping Us Hooked* (New York: Penguin Press, 2017).

218 Ibid., pg. 2.

219 Y. Y. Tang, et al., "Mindfulness meditation improves emotion regulation and reduces drug abuse," *Drug and Alcohol Dependence* 163, Suppl. 1 (2016): S13–8.

220 Y. Y. Tang, "Circuitry of self-control and its role in reducing addiction," *Trends in Cognitive Sciences* 19, no. 8 (2015): 439–44.

221 Y. Y. Tang, "Brief meditation training induces smoking reduction," *Proceedings of the National Academy of Sciences of the United States* 110, no. 34 (2013): 13971–75.

222 R. A. Gotink, et al., "8-week Mindfulness Based Stress Reduction induces brain changes similar to traditional long-term meditation practice–A systematic review," *Brain and Cognition* 108 (2016): 32–41.

223 www.health.harvard.edu/newsletter_article/napping-may-not-be-such-a-no-no.

224 Lopez-Guilera, et al., "CLOCK 3111 T/C SNP Interacts with Emotional Eating Behavior for Weight-Loss in a Mediterranean Population," *PLoS One* 9, (June 2014), 99–152.

225 A. O'Connor, How Sleep Loss Adds to Weight Gain, *New York Times* (August 6, 2013); *see also* A. J. Krauss, et al., "The Sleep-Deprived Human Brain," *Nature Reviews Neuroscience* 18 (2017): 404–18, *see also* S. R. Patel et al., "Association Between Reduced Sleep and Weight Gain in Women," *American Journal of Epidemiology* 164, no. 10 (2006): 947–54.

226 A. N. Goldstein-Piekarski, S. M. Greer, J. M. Saletin, M. P. Walker, "Sleep Deprivation Impairs the Human Central and Peripheral Nervous System Discrimination of Social Threat," *The Journal of Neuroscience* 35 (2015): 10135–45.

227 T. Horesh, "Drug Addicts and Their Music: A Story of a Complex Relationship," in *Music Therapy and Addictions* (Philadelphia, PA: Jessica Kingsley Publishers, 2012), 57.

228 Ibid.

229 L. Rivera, "Dancing Myself Into Recovery: The Benefits of Dance Movement Therapy," SoberRecovery, January 23, 2017, www.soberrecovery.com,

230 L. Goodison and H. Schafter, "Drug addiction therapy, A dance to the music of time," *The Health Sciences Journal* 109 (1999): 28–29; P. Muller, "Dancing or Fitness Sport? The Effects of Two Training Programs on Hippocampal Plasticity and Balance Abilities in Healthy Seniors," *Frontiers in Human Neuroscience* 11 (2017): 305.

231 C. De la Huerta, *Coming Out Spiritually: The Next Step* (New York: Penguin Putnam Books, 1999), 132.

CHAPTER TWELVE

232 M. S. Westerterp-Plantenga, *Protein Intake and Energy Balance.*

233 M. E. Bocarsly, L. A. Berner, B. G. Hoebel, N. M. Avena, "Rats that binge eat fat-rich food do not show somatic signs or anxiety associated with opiate-like withdrawal: implications for nutrient-specific food addiction behaviors," Physiology & Behavior, Princeton University (May 24, 2011).

234 Beasley and Knightly, *Food for Recovery*, 21.

235 Ibid., at Conclusion.

236 N. M. Avena, P. Rada, and B. G. Hoebel, "Evidence for sugar addiction: behavioral and neurochemical effects of intermittent, excessive sugar intake," *Neuroscience and Biobehavioral Reviews* 32, no. 1 (2008): 20–39.

237 F. Batmanghelidj, *Water: You're Not Sick, You're Thirsty*, (Woodland Hills, CA: Global Health Solutions, Inc., 2008), 16–17.

238 Ibid., *Water*, 58.

239 Naveed Sattar, G., Dr, *Fruit Juice, Just Another Sugary Drink?*, The Lancet Diabetes & Endocrinology, 2014.

240 M. G. Perri, S. D. Anton, P. E. Durning, T. U. Ketterson, S. J. Sydeman, N. E. Berlant, "Adherence to exercise prescriptions: effects of prescribing moderate versus higher levels of intensity and frequency," *Health Psychology* 21, no. 5 (2002): 452–58.

241 R. B. Kanarek, K. E. D'Anci, N. Jurdak, and W. F. Mathes, "Running and addiction: precipitated withdrawal in a rat model of activity-based anorexia," *Behavioral. Neuroscience* 123, no. 4 (2009): 905–12.

242 R. A. Brown, et al., "A Pilot Study of Aerobic Exercise as an Adjunctive Treatment for Drug Dependence," *Mental Health and Physical Activity* 3, no. 1 (2010): 27–34; Teen Athletes at Low Risk for Opioid Addiction, University of Michigan, Pediatrics, 2016).

243 C. Robertson, et al., "Effect of exercise training on striatal dopamine D2/D3 receptors in methamphetamine users during behavioral treatment," *Journal of Neuropsychopharmocology* 41, no. 6 (2015): 1629–36.

244 A. Byrne, D. G. Byrne, "The effect of exercise on depression, anxiety and other mood states: A review," *Journal of Psychosomatic Research* 37, no. 6 (1993): 565–74.

245 M. G. Calvo, "Anxiety and heart rate under psychological stress: The effects of exercise-training," *Anxiety, Stress, and Coping: An International Journal* 9, no. 4 (1996): 321–37.

246 T. R. Collingwood, et al., "Physical fitness effects on substance abuse risk factors and use patterns," *Journal of Drug Education* 21, no. 1 (1991): 73–84.

247 P. Ekkekakis, et al., "Walking in (affective) circles: Can short walks enhance affect?" *Journal of Behavioral Medicine* 23 (2000): 245–75.

248 The actual benefit depends on the intensity of the training. See *Does Exercise Raise Your Metabolic Rate for Several Hours After the Workout?* Michael Hutchins, February 7, 2014, www.livestrong.com/article/485498-does-exercise-raise-your-metabolic-rate-for-several-hours-after-the-workout.

249 L. Kaminoff and A. Matthews, *Yoga Anatomy, Your Illustrated Guide to Postures, Movements, and Breathing Techniques* (Leeds, UK: Human Kinetics Europe, Ltd., 2012).

CHAPTER FOURTEEN

250 W. Wilson, *The Twelve Steps and Twelve Traditions* (New York: Alcoholics Anonymous World Services), 89–90.

251 Ibid.

CHAPTER FIFTEEN

252 A. Terraneo, et al., "Transcranial magnetic stimulation of dorsolateral prefrontal cortex reduces cocaine use: A pilot study," *European Neuropsychopharmacology* 26, no. 1 (2016): 37–44.

253 K. Blum, et al., "The Molecular Neurobiology of Twelve Step Program & Fellowship: Connecting the Dots for Recovery," *Journal of Reward Deficiency Syndrome* 1, no. 1 (2015): 46–64.

254 Ibid.

255 A. R. Krentzman, "Gratitude, abstinence and alcohol use disorders: Report of a preliminary finding," *Journal of Substance Abuse Treatment* 78 (2017): 30–36.

256 Narcotics Anonymous, *Just For Today*, 236.